VIMAZI TRACK CLUB

Running in Circles

Sciencey, Gamey, Head-Scratchy Track Workouts for Faster Running

Scott Tucker & John Zilly
Illustrated by Jason Grube

Adventure Press

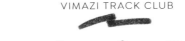

VIMAZI TRACK CLUB

Running in Circles
Sciencey, Gamey, Head-Scratchy
Track Workouts for Faster Running

The brains & the brawn (unsure which is which)

Don't try to "pop in" for a visit. Just sayin'...

Don't steal!

Adventure Press
PO Box 14059
Seattle, Washington 98114

All lefts are o.k. though

Illustrator: Jason Grube
Copy Editor: Avra Dolan

adventurepress.com
vimazi.com

Adequate with a pencil.

CLICK HERE for awesomeness!

She's makes the words so good with the edits

ISBN 978-1-881583-13-4

Disclaimer: The authors have taken great care in dreaming up, run-testing, and writing each of these workouts. If you get confused partway through a workout, they strenuously disclaim any and all responsibility. Furthermore, running intervals is by definition a stressful endeavor; it's your responsibility to make sure you have sufficient fitness before running any of these workouts. Let's bring this down the homestretch to say that the authors, publisher, and FastEquation are in no way responsible for any running problems you may have or encounter, physical or otherwise, from use of this book.

Claimer: If, on the other hand, you find great joy within the pages of this book and become a faster runner because of it, the authors happily take full responsibility.

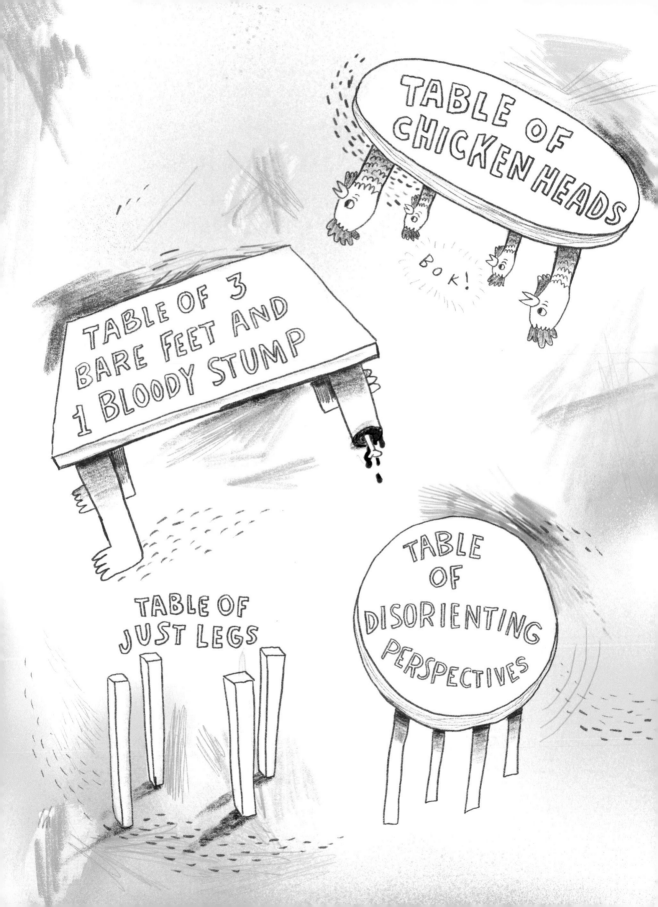

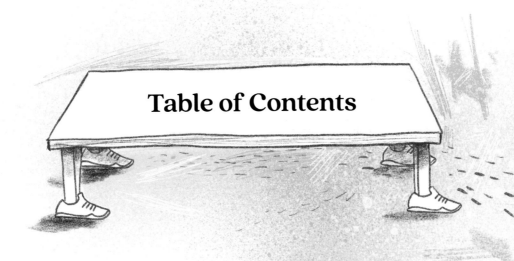

Table of Contents

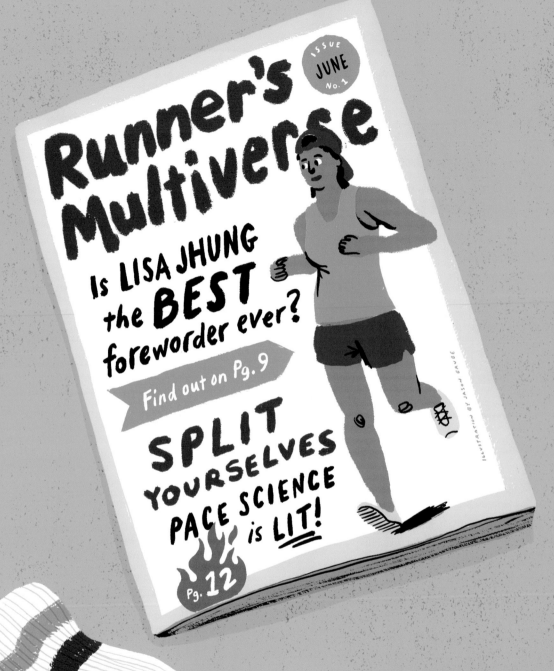

Less Dreckery, More Creativity

These guys I sort of know asked me to write a foreword for their new book. Flattered? Of course. But why me? Well, their book and my latest book, *Running That Doesn't Suck: How to Love Running (Even if You Think You Hate It)*, aren't completely unrelated. Both set out to mix some literal and figurative color into the conventional running book bookshelves.

I've been in the running industry a long time. About 100 years ago, I was an editor at *Trail Runner* magazine. After that I co-founded *Adventure Sports* magazine. And after that, I was a contributing editor to *Runner's World* and freelance writer. Along the way, I blogged about being a pregnant runner, managed a trail running website, wrote a shoes and gear blog, and sweated out a lot of gear reviews, profiles, race stories, and so on. I currently write about running for a range of publications, including *Outside*. All to say that I've written and edited a lot of running content over the years. If you're not careful, running stories and advice (like running, like anything!) can get repetitive.

Then these two guys—John Zilly and Scott Tucker—shared a book concept with me. I thought, "Hmm, maybe interesting." When they shared the illustrations, title, and some write-ups for the workouts, surely I cracked a sly grin. I was actually sold by just the illustrations ... the fact that there even *are* illustrations, and artistic, ridiculously conceptual ones at that. My books are conceptually illustrated too, but these got me.

I was inspired and fired up. Not just by a running book with great workouts that will make us all as fast as cheetahs, but with the sheer creativity that went into it. The workouts are creative. The storytelling is creative. The illustrations are, insanely and undeniably, creative. In a world where way too much information is thrown at us in exponentially more boring and conventional ways, TRUE CREATIVITY IS A FANTASTIC THING. This book inspires me to not only get out to the track more often for good, fun, ass-kicking interval workouts, it has inspired me to push boundaries of creative thinking in all parts of my life. To me, that is the definition of inspiration.

So, enjoy this collection of "Sciencey, Gamey, Head-Scratchy Track Workouts." And may your running—along with every other aspect of your life—be inspired.

LISA JHUNG
Author of *Running That Doesn't Suck: How to Love Running (Even If You Think You Hate It)* and *Trailhead: The Dirt on All Things Trail Running*

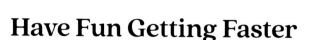
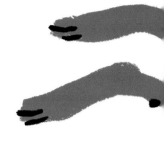

Have Fun Getting Faster

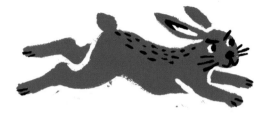

HAVE FUN

We've held weekly 5:45 a.m. Vimazi Track Club interval workouts for a long time. To keep them engaging and memorable, we come up with a theme that animates each session. Why? Track workouts have a reputation for being tedious, repetitive, boring, and dull. We think life should be tasty and full of curiosities, and track workouts shouldn't be any different. You might as well enjoy a story, a puzzle, or a sciencey confection while you run your guts out.

Intervals can make your lungs burn and your muscles quiver, and there's something darkly, runnerishly funny about that. So in addition to a think-and-run-at-the-same-time theme, we've tried to tap into a small keg of rogue humor. We hope these workouts are as entertaining to peruse and select as they are energizing to run. Each has been scientifically informed by current best practices, has its own sugary rhythm, and has been fully track-tested.

GET FAST

Whatever you think about intervals, there's zero question about their efficacy. They'll make you a faster runner. You'll also improve your form and learn how to push harder during a race. Getting faster takes some time, but the results of track work will surprise you. We recommend one interval workout a week, especially during the buildup to a race.

Track intervals that work on speed are one of the four basic elements of any good training program. **Endurance** builds a bigger fuel tank so you can run farther. **Economy** builds a more fuel-efficient engine so you can maintain a pace with less effort. **Resilience** builds your entire body's ability to handle training without breaking down. **Speed** builds horsepower so you can run faster over longer distances.

SELECT A WORKOUT

We run distance at Vimazi Track Club, so these workouts are intended to help improve race times at distances of 5k and farther. Especially farther.

We've separated this book into three sections—longish, mediumish, and shortish (a somewhat loose classification system). Selecting a workout is all about your training objective. Early in your race buildup, you probably want to focus on longish intervals. They'll help with consistent pacing and maintaining speed during a race. Move to mediumish and shortish intervals as your event gets closer. These will help increase your anaerobic threshold and get you more comfortable with a quick turnover. Both will lead to a faster pace and a better finish time.

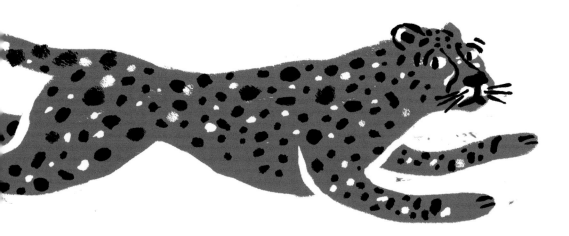

Don't let longish, mediumish, and shortish designations give you the wrong idea. Each of these workouts is essentially the same length, give or take a few hundred meters. They all include about 8000 meters of intensity running (20 laps on a 400m track or essentially 5 miles). Why 8000 meters? That's the sweet spot for most serious runners. Pros and sub-elites may occasionally run longer; free spirits may want to run a shorter total distance. We didn't think total length should be an added decision variable when selecting a workout.

Be sure to note the difficulty rating. We've calculated it using the flaming lung methodology. The Lung Burn for each workout is measured from one to five, five being complete immolation. The shortish intervals tend to be the toughest because they have the most fast-paced running.

RUN THE WORKOUT

We've based most of the interval speeds on your 5k and 10k race paces. Find your corresponding lap and multi-lap paces on the pacing cheat sheet, page 12. If you don't have a recent race time to work from, think of it this way: 10K pace is hard, 5K pace is very hard, and a sprint leaves you breathless.

Warming up for at least 15–20 minutes is the best way to hit your target interval paces (don't forget a 10–20 minutes of cool down). Note that running

injuries are common, so stretch, warm up, and if you're new to intervals don't overdo your first day on the track. Strides are a nice warmup: Alternate 20–30 seconds of high cadence running with 30 seconds of easy jogging over 800m. Strides should make you feel light and agile.

Almost all the rest periods should be active, which means you jog them. No hands-on-knees gasping! Some of the rests are only 10 seconds or simply a change of pace.

If your training plan calls for 10 miles on track day, work the additional 5 miles into a warmup and cool down. Or run two separate workouts. If your plan calls for fewer than 6 miles, keep the workout's rhythm and objective by removing intervals rather than decreasing interval distances. Don't skimp on the warmup or cool down.

FIND YOUR PACE

These workouts are meant to help you reach your optimal pace. In distance running, pace is your superpower, so tap into it. While you might decide to take our commentary — the hurt, the pain, the soul-crushing piles of quivering Jell-O — with a grain of salt, we're pretty sure we mean every word, in a runner's dark humor sort of way. Our hope is that these intervals will inspire a love for track workouts and a thirst to run faster.

Pacing Cheat Sheet

	RACE TIMES			SPLIT TIMES				
Mile	5k	10k	400m	800m	1200m	1600m	2000m	3200m
04:01	12:30	25:00	01:00	02:00	03:00	04:00	05:00	08:00
04:09	12:55	25:50	01:02	02:04	03:06	04:08	05:10	08:16
04:17	13:20	26:40	01:04	02:08	03:12	04:16	05:20	08:32
04:26	13:45	27:30	01:06	02:12	03:18	04:24	05:30	08:48
04:34	14:10	28:20	01:08	02:16	03:24	04:32	05:40	09:04
04:42	14:35	29:10	01:10	02:20	03:30	04:40	05:50	09:20
04:50	15:00	30:00	01:12	02:24	03:36	04:48	06:00	09:36
04:58	15:25	30:50	01:14	02:28	03:42	04:56	06:10	09:52
05:06	15:50	31:40	01:16	02:32	03:48	05:04	06:20	10:08
05:14	16:15	32:30	01:18	02:36	03:54	05:12	06:30	10:24
05:22	16:40	33:20	01:20	02:40	04:00	05:20	06:40	10:40
05:30	17:05	34:10	01:22	02:44	04:06	05:28	06:50	10:56
05:38	17:30	35:00	01:24	02:48	04:12	05:36	07:00	11:12
05:46	17:55	35:50	01:26	02:52	04:18	05:44	07:10	11:28
05:54	18:20	36:40	01:28	02:56	04:24	05:52	07:20	11:44
06:02	18:45	37:30	01:30	03:00	04:30	06:00	07:30	12:00
06:10	19:10	38:20	01:32	03:04	04:36	06:08	07:40	12:16
06:18	19:35	39:10	01:34	03:08	04:42	06:16	07:50	12:32
06:26	20:00	40:00	01:36	03:12	04:48	06:24	08:00	12:48
06:34	20:25	40:50	01:38	03:16	04:54	06:32	08:10	13:04
06:42	20:50	41:40	01:40	03:20	05:00	06:40	08:20	13:20
06:50	21:15	42:30	01:42	03:24	05:06	06:48	08:30	13:36
06:58	21:40	43:20	01:44	03:28	05:12	06:56	08:40	13:52
07:06	22:05	44:10	01:46	03:32	05:18	07:04	08:50	14:08
07:15	22:30	45:00	01:48	03:36	05:24	07:12	09:00	14:24
07:23	22:55	45:50	01:50	03:40	05:30	07:20	09:10	14:40
07:31	23:20	46:40	01:52	03:44	05:36	07:28	09:20	14:56
07:39	23:45	47:30	01:54	03:48	05:42	07:36	09:30	15:12
07:47	24:10	48:20	01:56	03:52	05:48	07:44	09:40	15:28
07:55	24:35	49:10	01:58	03:56	05:54	07:52	09:50	15:44
08:03	25:00	50:00	02:00	04:00	06:00	08:00	10:00	16:00

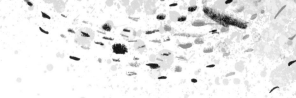

RACE TIMES				SPLIT TIMES					
Mile	**5k**	**10k**	**400m**	**800m**	**1200m**	**1600m**	**2000m**	**3200m**
08:11	25:25	50:50	02:02	04:04	06:06	08:08	10:10	16:16
08:19	25:50	51:40	02:04	04:08	06:12	08:16	10:20	16:32
08:27	26:15	52:30	02:06	04:12	06:18	08:24	10:30	16:48
08:35	26:40	53:20	02:08	04:16	06:24	08:32	10:40	17:04
08:43	27:05	54:10	02:10	04:20	06:30	08:40	10:50	17:20
08:51	27:30	55:00	02:12	04:24	06:36	08:48	11:00	17:36
08:59	27:55	55:50	02:14	04:28	06:42	08:56	11:10	17:52
09:07	28:20	56:40	02:16	04:32	06:48	09:04	11:20	18:08
09:15	28:45	57:30	02:18	04:36	06:54	09:12	11:30	18:24
09:23	29:10	58:20	02:20	04:40	07:00	09:20	11:40	18:40
09:31	29:35	59:10	02:22	04:44	07:06	09:28	11:50	18:56
09:39	30:00	60:00	02:24	04:48	07:12	09:36	12:00	19:12
09:47	30:25	60:50	02:26	04:52	07:18	09:44	12:10	19:28
09:55	30:50	61:40	02:28	04:56	07:24	09:52	12:20	19:44
10:04	31:15	62:30	02:30	05:00	07:30	10:00	12:30	20:00
10:12	31:40	63:20	02:32	05:04	07:36	10:08	12:40	20:16
10:20	32:05	64:10	02:34	05:08	07:42	10:16	12:50	20:32
10:28	32:30	65:00	02:36	05:12	07:48	10:24	13:00	20:48
10:36	32:55	65:50	02:38	05:16	07:54	10:32	13:10	21:04
10:44	33:20	66:40	02:40	05:20	08:00	10:40	13:20	21:20
10:52	33:45	67:30	02:42	05:24	08:06	10:48	13:30	21:36
11:00	34:10	68:20	02:44	05:28	08:12	10:56	13:40	21:52
11:08	34:35	69:10	02:46	05:32	08:18	11:04	13:50	22:08
11:16	35:00	70:00	02:48	05:36	08:24	11:12	14:00	22:24
11:24	35:25	70:50	02:50	05:40	08:30	11:20	14:10	22:40
11:32	35:50	71:40	02:52	05:44	08:36	11:28	14:20	22:56
11:40	36:15	72:30	02:54	05:48	08:42	11:36	14:30	23:12
11:48	36:40	73:20	02:56	05:52	08:48	11:44	14:40	23:28
11:56	37:05	74:10	02:58	05:56	08:54	11:52	14:50	23:44
12:04	37:30	75:00	03:00	06:00	09:00	12:00	15:00	24:00

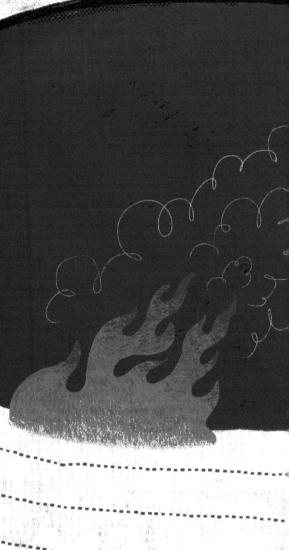

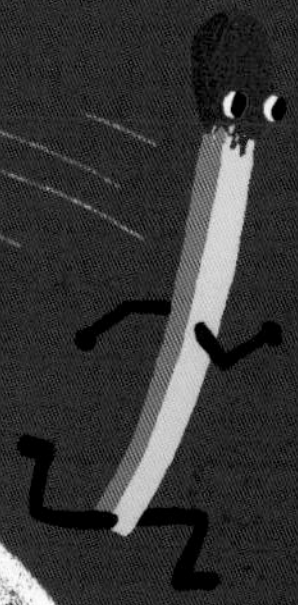

MEMORIZING PI

WORD GAMES

LIMERICK CHALLENGE

PULL A LANDY

GÖDEL'S PARADOX

ENTANGLED WORLDS

BEWARE THE PTERODACTYL

TRACK THE ZODIAC

BIGHORN SPIRALS

GEOMETRY FREAKOUT

INTERVALS

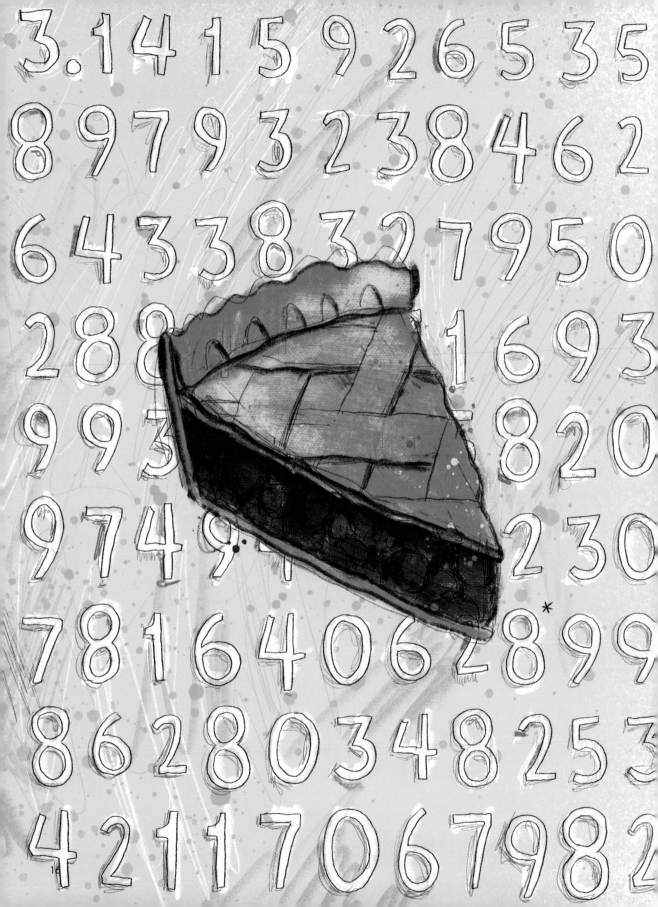

Memorizing Pi

PIE! PIE! PIE!

DISTANCES: 1200, 400, 1600, 400, 2000, 2400

- -

LUNG BURN: 🔥

Pi is what's called an irrational number, meaning it can't be written as a fraction. In simple terms, it's defined as the ratio of a circle's circumference to its diameter. But you'll find pi in all sorts of complex mathematical formulas and physics equations. Ancient Egyptian, Greek, Chinese, and Indian mathematicians all developed fairly accurate ways to calculate pi, mostly so buildings and bridges wouldn't fall down.

If you took geometry and were exceedingly lucky, you may have been required to memorize just the first few digits of pi. 3.14159 sound familiar? More than likely, knowing those six digits has had zero impact on your life other than taking up neural space that could have been used for something important, like actual pie recipes. May we suggest strawberry rhubarb?

HOW TO RUN IT

Starting with the 3, each digit in pi represents an interval. The numeral determines the number of laps in each interval. Therefore, for the first interval, you'll run a 1200 because 3 x 400 = 1200. Don't worry, you're only running six digits out, and we'll cheat a bit by changing the 9 to a 6 (the ancients would certainly object!) to limit this workout to our self-imposed 8000 meters. For pacing, run the 400s faster than your 5k pace, and run the longer intervals at your 10k pace.

REST INTERVAL

60-second active rest between intervals

HERE'S WHERE IT HURTS

If you're not sufficiently warmed up, it may be tough to catch your breath during the first 400. But maintaining focus during the fourth and fifth laps of the final interval will likely be where you start choking on numbers.

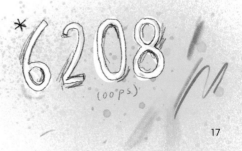

*6208
(oops)

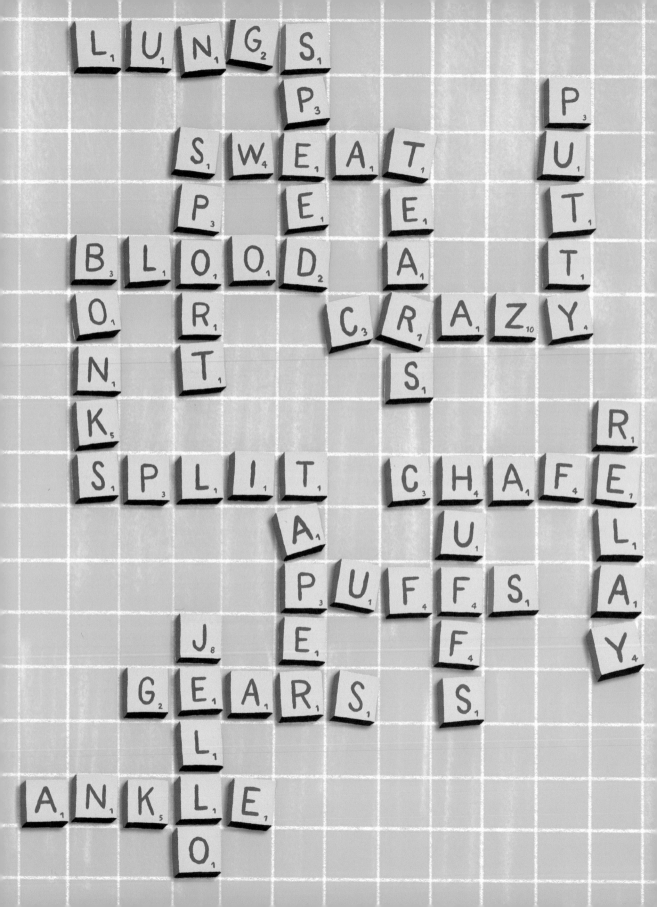

Word Games

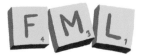

DISTANCES: 400, 800, 1200, 1600, 2000, 2000

- -

LUNG BURN:

How did language develop? Theories abound! The Pooh-Pooh Theory suggests it comes from the sounds we make in response to pain, surprise, or bad smells. Bow-Wow theorists say we like to mimic the sounds we hear. According to the Yo-He-Ho Theory, language is derived from the grunts of physical labor. The La-La Theory supposes that humming, chanting, playfulness, and love sparked language. Ancient runners likely played their roles: the stinky loincloths, the easily mimicked footstrikes, the grunting on hill repeats, and the joyous hum of easy running.

For today's Board-Game Theory, you'll build a five-letter word—letter by letter for each of the first five intervals. You get your first letter, preferably randomly selected by a teammate, after the 400. For each successive interval, carefully choose a letter to add on to the ones you've already collected. The catch: Every time you add a letter, the result must be a new word. Example: If you get a *b* for your first interval, you might build these four words: second interval—*be*, third—*bee*, fourth—*beet*, fifth—*beets*. If you get stuck building your word (and intermediate words) and need to rearrange or exchange letters, run the entire next interval faster than your 5k pace.

HOW TO RUN IT

Run your consonant laps at your 10k pace. Run your vowel laps faster than your 5k pace (vowels are handy, so they hurt a little more). Notice you add a lap for each new letter you accumulate: 400, 800, 1200, etc. The final 2000—you're done building words—is a mind-clearing speed progression. Starting in lane 5, run each lap faster than the previous one. Move inward with each lap to finish in lane 1. Be grateful the game doesn't go to six letters.

REST INTERVAL

60- to 90-second active rest between intervals

HERE'S WHERE IT HURTS

As you run, your leg muscles will gradually deprive your brain of oxygen. Spelling short words becomes labored, and coherent thoughts break into fragments. Your language will devolve from pleasant La-Las to gasping grunts.

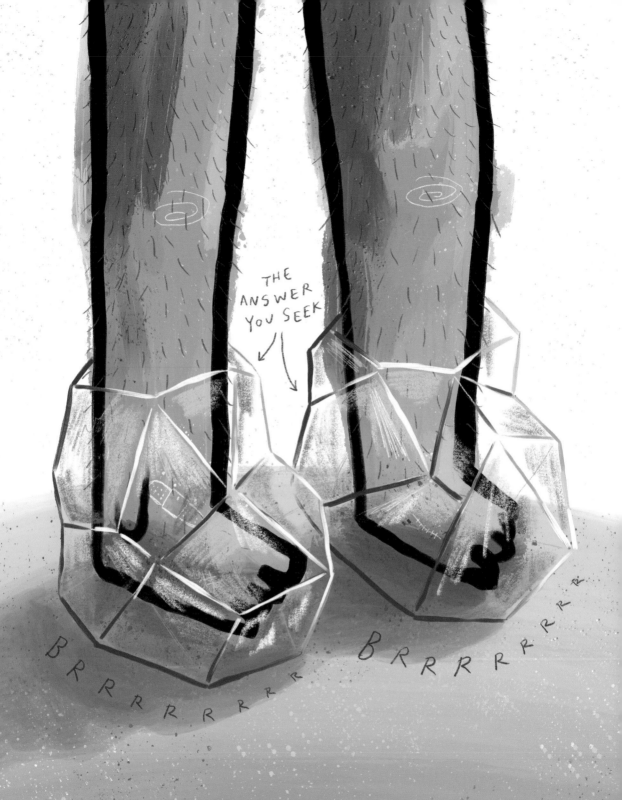

Limerick Challenge

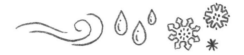

DISTANCES: 5 x 1600

- -

LUNG BURN:

Peter Sagal, avid runner and author of *The Incomplete Book of Running*, hosts the NPR show *Wait Wait… Don't Tell Me!* During the Listener Limerick Challenge each week, announcer Bill Kurtis reads limericks written by Philipp Goedicke. Listeners and one lucky contestant must guess the last word of each limerick. So here's our limerick:

As you run through cold rain and hard sleet,
Are you longing for summer's dry heat?
Those bright shirtless days?
And warm sunny rays?
Too bad, now's time to suffer cold _____.

HOW TO RUN IT

Five lines to a limerick results in five intervals (I mean, duh!). Since limericks follow an AABBA rhyming pattern, run the first lap of intervals 1, 2, and 5 slightly faster than your 5k pace. For intervals 3 and 4, run the last lap sub 5k pace. Run all other laps at your 10k pace.

REST INTERVAL

60-second active rest between intervals

HERE'S WHERE IT HURTS

Buckle down for these mile repeats.
Five laps extra hard, what a feat!
But of course you should know
That the faster you go
Makes the fifth mile quite hard to _____.

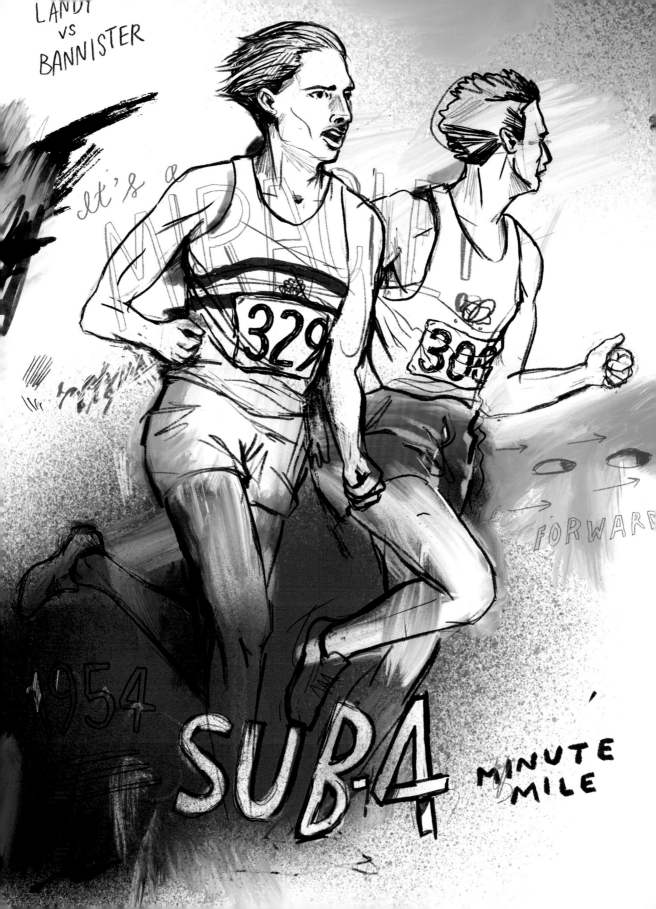

Pull a Landy

KEEP YOUR EYES ON THE PRIZE

DISTANCES: 5 x 1600

- -

LUNG BURN:

Middle-distance runner John Landy is probably best known for a race he lost. On August 7, 1954, Landy, an Australian, ran a much-anticipated duel against Roger Bannister of Britain at the Commonwealth Games in Vancouver, B.C., a race sometimes called the Miracle Mile.

In May of that year, Bannister ran the first ever sub-4-minute mile (3:59.4). Just six weeks later, Landy broke Bannister's world record with a 3:57.9. In the Commonwealth Games race, listened to over the radio by an estimated 100 million people, Landy led the first three laps, with Bannister a close second. As they rounded the final turn, Landy looked over his left shoulder to see where his competitor was. Bannister, however, had moved to the outside and kicked passed Landy on the right. Bannister won in 3:58.8 due in part to Landy's poorly timed glance.

HOW TO RUN IT

Run each 1600 at your 5k pace, but lengthen the finishing sprint on each subsequent interval. Sprint the final 100m of the first 1600, the final 200m of your second, and so on until sprinting the final 500m of your fifth interval. But your interval doesn't count unless you look over your left shoulder as you begin each sprint.

REST INTERVAL

2-minute active rest between intervals

HERE'S WHERE IT HURTS

Let's face it, leaning in to ever-longer sprints as you go deeper into mile repeats isn't easy. You'll accumulate a whole lot of suffer points during the fourth and fifth 1600s, especially on the final laps. That said, looking over your left shoulder before each of those sprints, knowing a Bannister-like figure is fated to pass you, adds a heavy psychic weight to the hurt.

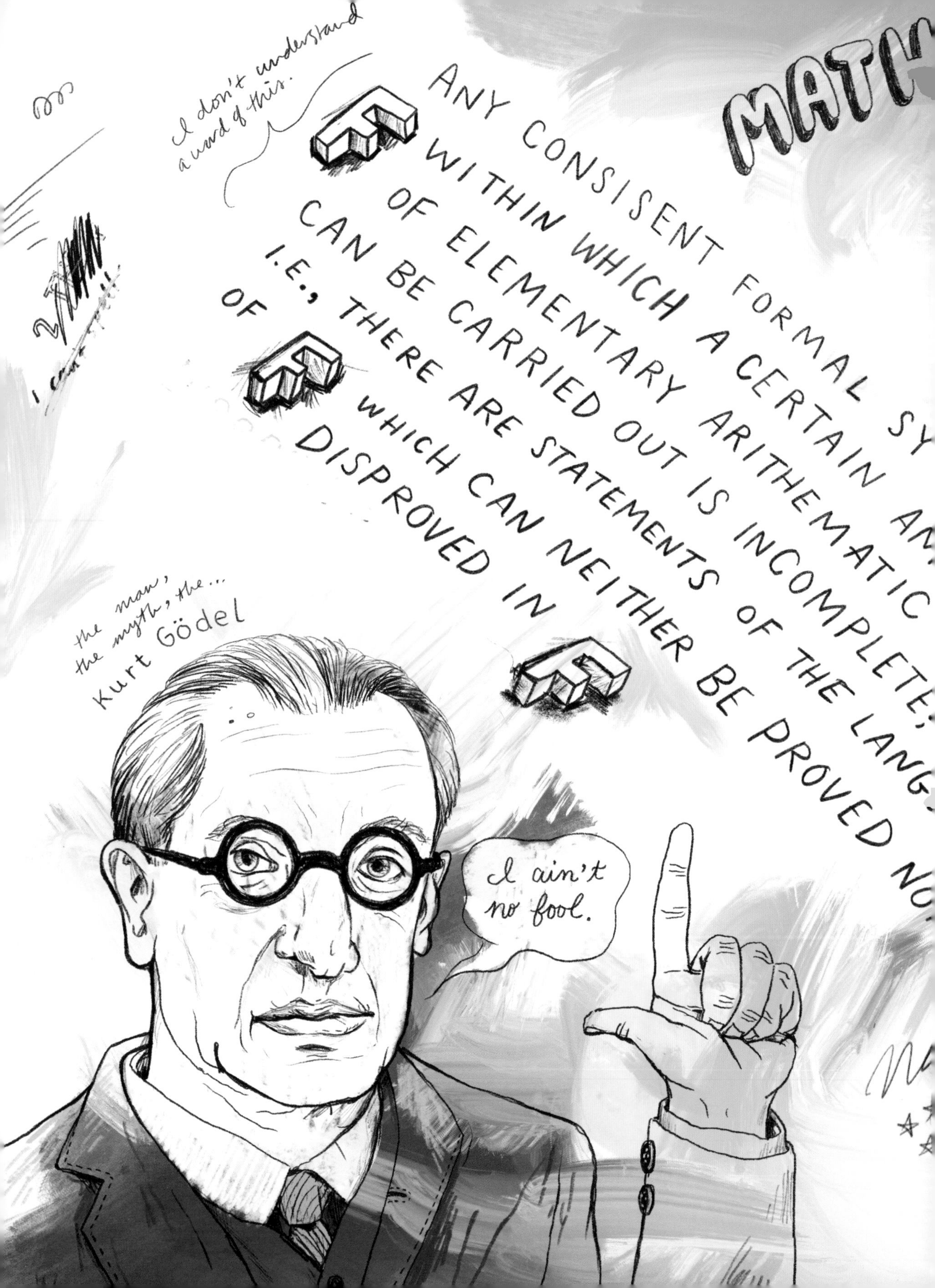
MATH
I don't understand a word of this.
ANY CONSISENT FORMAL SY
WITHIN WHICH A CERTAIN AM
OF ELEMENTARY ARITHEMATIC
CAN BE CARRIED OUT IS INCOMPLETE;
I.E., THERE ARE STATEMENTS OF THE LANG
OF WHICH CAN NEITHER BE PROVED NO
DISPROVED IN
the man, the myth, the...
Kurt Gödel
I ain't no fool.

Gödel's Paradox

This statement is false

DISTANCES: 1600, 3600, 800, 2000

- -

LUNG BURN:

Mathematician and analytic philosopher Kurt Gödel, 1906–1978, is up there with Aristotle as one of the most influential logicians ever. In one instance of his complete badassness, he pioneered a process of encoding known as Gödel numbering. (Don't worry, we won't get into it.)

In 1931, at age 25, Gödel published not one but two *incompleteness theorems.* In a formal mathematical system, these theorems posited there must be at least one true but unprovable statement. If all statements were provable, the system would necessarily be false. Cue exploding head. These theorems led to Gödel's famous paradox: *This statement is false.* Go ahead and analyze all you want, but one statement is true: We're going to use Gödel's paradox to run intervals.

HOW TO RUN IT

Each word in *this statement is false* represents an interval, and each letter equals one lap. Run the consonants at your 10k pace and the vowels at your 5k pace.

REST INTERVAL

90-second active rest between intervals

HERE'S WHERE IT HURTS

With three vowels in the word *statement,* your 3600 will take a toll so long as you complete it. Analytically speaking, the *l* and *s* in *false* aren't too friendly either.

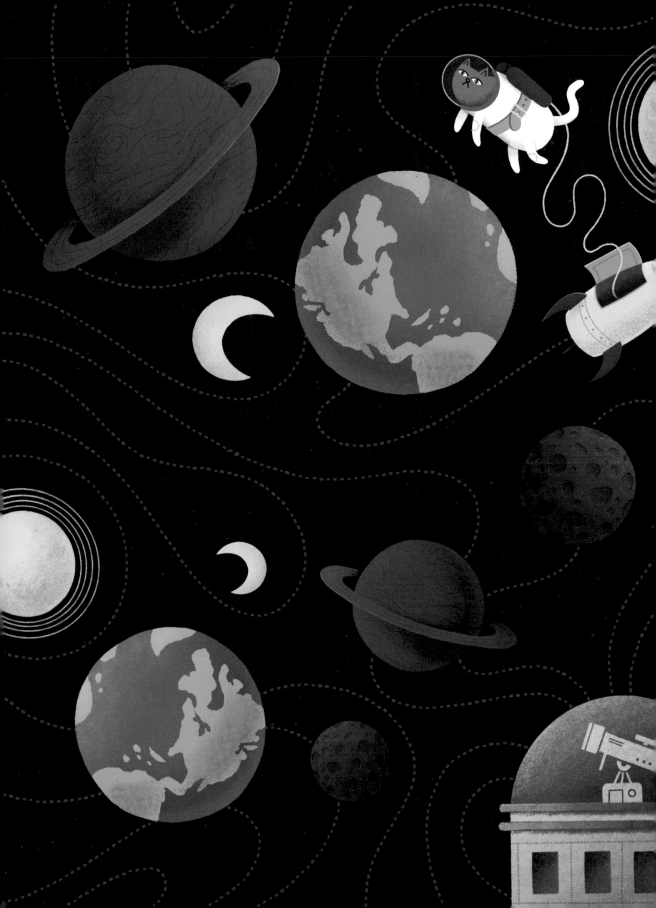

Entangled Worlds

DISTANCES: 5 × 1600

- -

LUNG BURN: 🔥 🔥 🔥

In honor of *Something Deeply Hidden* by Sean Carroll, as well as the works of other theoretical physicists like Hugh Everett and Bryce DeWitt, this workout pays tribute to the many-worlds interpretation of quantum mechanics. (You may come to call it many-miles.) According to the many-worlds interpretation, particles are entangled with each other and are governed by the one and only universal wave function. Things get weirder with a process called quantum decoherence: When a quantum system interacts with its environment, the universe branches into two copies. So it's true—probability is an illusion!

In the world of a 400m oval, you and another runner represent two entangled particles: You run the same speed but in opposite directions around the track. Each time you interact (every 200m if you're running the same speed), the universe branches, causing you and your counter-particle to move out one lane. Since we're also accounting for the Schrödinger equation, the intervals undulate in intensity.

HOW TO RUN IT

Pair up (entangle) with a runner of about the same speed. Start out running opposite directions in lane 1. As you pass each other about halfway around the track, interact by slapping hands. As a result of decoherence and branching, you both move out to lane 2. When you pass again at the end of 400m, move out to lane 3. Continue moving out as you pass and slap hands every 200m. Here's how the intensity undulates: Run even-lane laps faster than your 5k pace and odd-lane laps at your 10k pace.

REST INTERVAL

60- to 90-second active rest between intervals with your partner particle

HERE'S WHERE IT HURTS

Mile repeats take their toll by the end, and even the best sighted among us will begin seeing double. Beware, especially, the even-numbered lanes during your last two intervals.

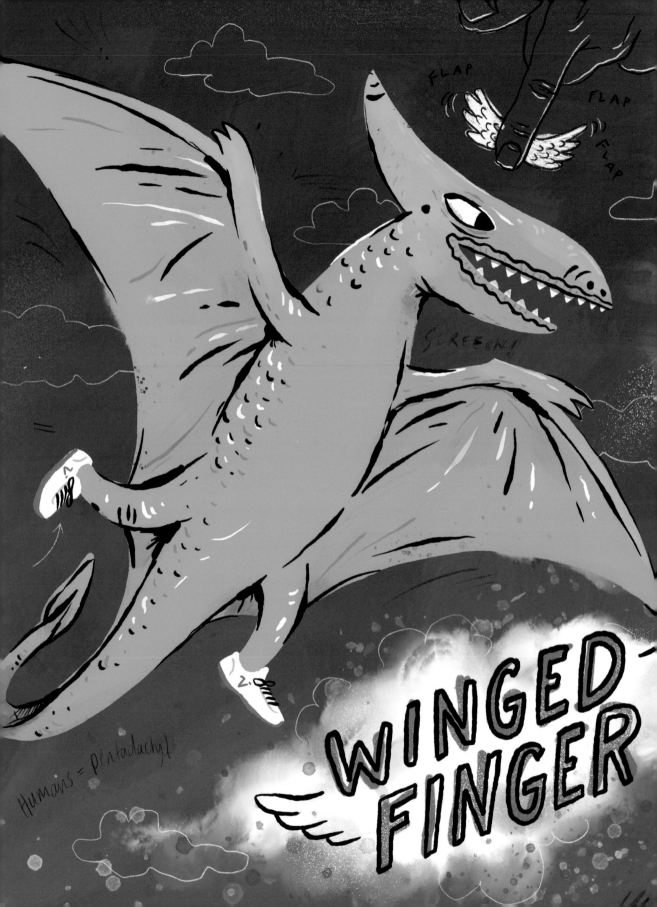

Beware the Pterodactyl

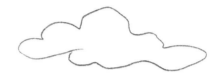

DISTANCES: 4 x 2000

- -

LUNG BURN:

A large flying reptile from the late Jurassic, and something to run away from (obvi!), *pterodactyl* literally means winged finger. So let's talk fingers, because you'll need them for counting. Humans are *pentadactyl*, which means five-fingered. Birds are *tetradactyl*, with three toes pointing forward and one pointing back for a total of four and perhaps an evolutionary just in case. With three fingers, the sloth rocks *tridactyl* digitry—something to know on days you don't feel like getting off the couch. Ostriches are *didactyl*. And horses are *monodactyl*. Monodactyl, incidentally, is how we feel at mile 22 of a marathon.

Okay, so imagine you're a small two-legged reptile out for a brisk run. Suddenly, a pterodactyl shadow looms over you. Adrenaline surges through your pentadactyl veins, and you run for your life. Once the danger passes, the brisk run continues.

HOW TO RUN IT

For each interval, run 4 of the 5 laps at your 10k pace and 1 of the 5 laps a bit faster than your 5k pace. Here's where you need your fingers for counting. Your over-threshold pterodactyl escape is the Human Lap (5th) for your first 2000, the Bird Lap (4th) for the second interval, the Sloth Lap (3rd) for the third interval, and the Ostrich Lap (2th) for the final interval.

REST INTERVAL

60-second active rest between intervals

HERE'S WHERE IT HURTS

Given the adrenaline rush of running from a pterodactyl, your fast lap isn't what really hurts. It's the subsequent lap that painfully reminds you: You're just a lowly reptile after all.

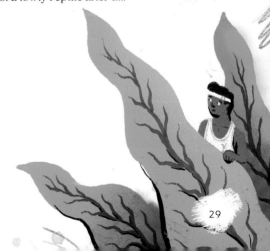

29

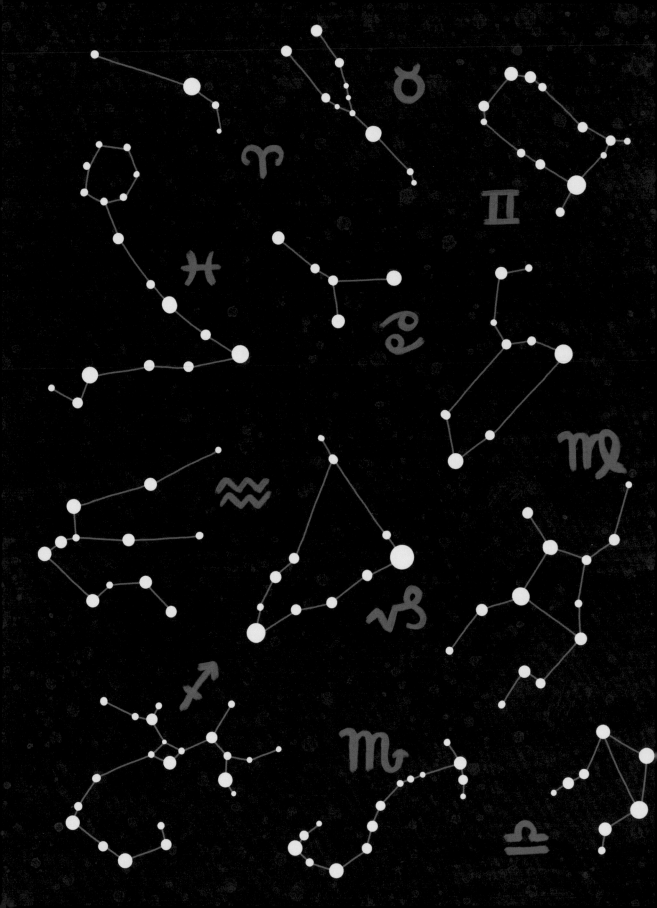

Track the Zodiac

DISTANCES: 1200, 5 x 500, 1200, 7 x 500

- -

LUNG BURN:

Bringing East and West together, this workout borrows from both the Chinese and Western zodiac. The Chinese zodiac follows a cycle of 12 years, the time it takes Jupiter to orbit the Sun. A different animal represents each of the 12 years. The word zodiac, by the way, comes from a Greek term meaning circle of animals. Each animal in the Chinese zodiac has a character influenced by, among other things, five natural elements: fire, water, earth, wood, and metal.

Meanwhile, the Western zodiac has 12 signs based on the 12 traditional constellations. The character of the signs is influenced by the five planets visible to the naked eye—Mercury, Venus, Mars, Saturn, Jupiter—plus the Sun and Moon. (Um, can you see fives, sevens, and twelves in your workout future?) A quick glance at the distances and this looks like a moderate workout. But read ahead, and you'll learn the sets of 500s are essentially extended intervals. Five characters for you: O-u-c-h-!

HOW TO RUN IT

Run the 1200s (for the 12 years and the 12 constellations) at your 10k pace. Run the 500s (which represent the 5 natural elements in the first set and 7 celestial bodies in the second) without rest, alternating your speed between slightly faster than your 10k pace to slightly faster than your 5k pace. Start the 500s in lane 5 and shift inward, adjusting your pace with each shift.

REST INTERVAL

60-second active rest after each 1200;
no rest between the 500s, just a change in intensity

HERE'S WHERE IT HURTS

Your Saturn will return numerous times while you shift from faster to slower to faster again during your last set of 500s. The real struggle could be remembering where each 500 ends. It may feel like searching for lost stars in the night sky.

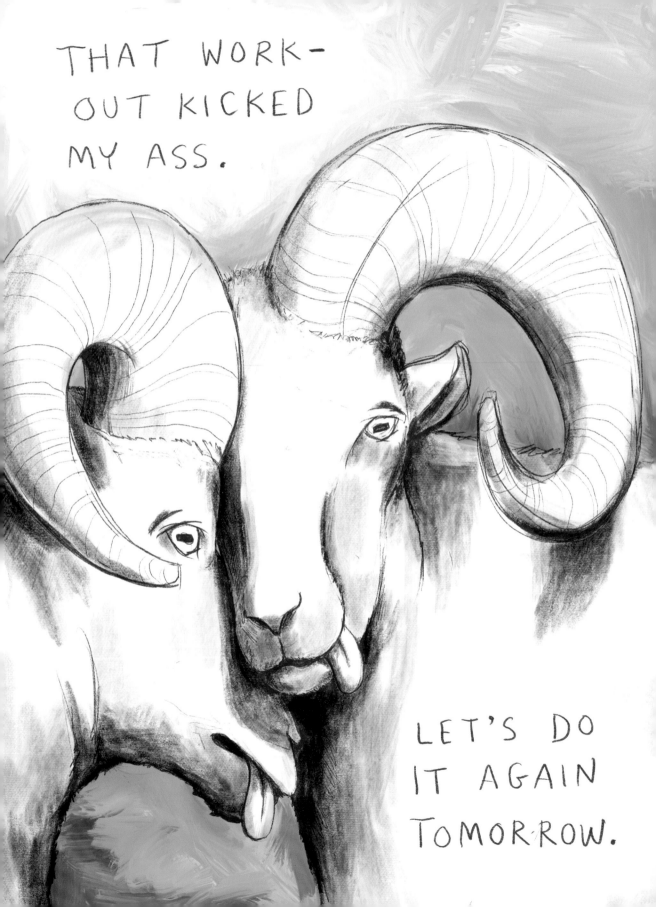

Bighorn Spirals

BAAAAAARF!

DISTANCES: 2 x 4000

- -

LUNG BURN:

Bighorn sheep enjoy roaming the meadows and craggy mountainsides of the Cascades, Sierra Nevadas, and Rockies, as well as the high deserts of the Southwest. Long ago, warming our long-distance runner hearts, these sheep trotted their way from Siberia to North America across the Bering land bridge. We'll call them ultrasheep and leave it at that.

As for the bighorn's most prominent attribute, the ewes have large horns with a slight curve; the rams sport thick, spiral horns. Turns out those ram horns can weigh up to 30 pounds, a hefty weight penalty if you've got an ultra planned anytime soon. Like idiotic males of all species, bighorn rams can't help themselves from fighting with other males. Horns are the weapon of choice as they repeatedly butt heads, usually during rut (mating season). For today, rather than fighting, we'll use the spiraling shape of the rams' horns to craft our workout. Now if we could only get a fitness tracker on those rams to track heart rate, steps, and elevation.

HOW TO RUN IT

Start this workout way out in lane 8. Sprint the first 200m, then settle into your 10k pace. At the end of the first lap, move into lane 7. Move in one lane after each lap; sprint the first 200m of each even-numbered lane. After running a lap in lane 1, move outward until you finish a lap in lane 3. Rest! For the second interval, begin in lane 3, move inward then back out until you complete a lap in lane 8, remembering to sprint the first 200m of every even-numbered lane.

REST INTERVAL

2-minute active rest between intervals

HERE'S WHERE IT HURTS

To be master of the obvious, this workout has you running 5 miles—with only one short break—at your 6-mile race pace. Furthermore, you are sprinting ten 200s. It's subtle, it won't destroy you like some workouts, and it's only rated two burning lungs, but it may kick your ass to the point you need smelling salts by the end.

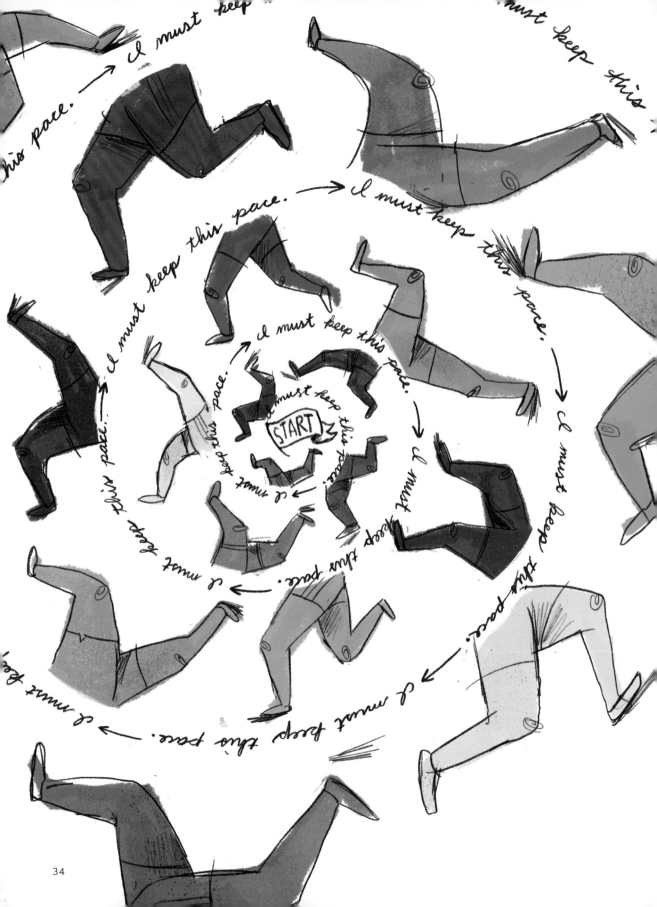

34

Geometry Freakout

DISTANCES: 1600, 2000, 1200, 1600, 1600

- -

LUNG BURN: 🔥 🔥 🔥

On Episode 391 of the popular *Freakonomics Radio* podcast, Steven Levitt mentions a survey that suggests fewer than 4% of American adults ever use geometry. As track runners, we're well versed in the oval-like 400m track. But let's expand our knowledge of geometric shapes. Spirals, like certain seashells, can be described mathematically by the rate a point moves away from the center as it goes around. An Archimedean spiral moves out at a constant rate. A Fibonacci spiral follows the Fibonacci sequence. A Hyperbolic spiral involves rapid exponential expansion. A Logarithmic spiral starts slowly then expands rapidly.

We'll utilize these different types of spirals to inflict ever-increasing pain. How, you ask? During each interval, you'll start in lane 1 then move outward according to the type of spiral. The catch is that every lap should clock in at the same time. And even a geometric simpleton knows that you run farther in lane 8 than lane 1.

HOW TO RUN IT

Start this workout at your 10k pace for lane 1. The sequence for your first Archimedean interval goes like this: lanes 1, 2, 3, 4. The second is Fibonacci: lanes 1, 1, 2, 3, 5. The third, Hyperbolic: lanes 1, 3, 8. For the fourth, run a Logarithmic spiral: lanes 1, 1½, 3, 8. For your fifth interval, run a reverse Archimedean: lanes 4, 3, 2, 1. The goal is to run even splits, even as you spiral into the outer lanes.

REST INTERVAL

60-second active rest between intervals

HERE'S WHERE IT HURTS

This is a tough workout, which you'll understand exquisitely during the last lap of your Hyperbolic and Logarithmic intervals. But the work to fine-tune your pace and remember what lane to run in might prove the most challenging.

MEDIUMISH

FIBONACCI

VACATION TO MERCURY

PALINDROME

BETELGEUSE

TOUR DE HURT

CHERRY BLOSSOMS

RUN YOUR SCALES

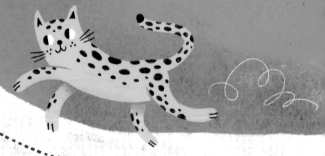

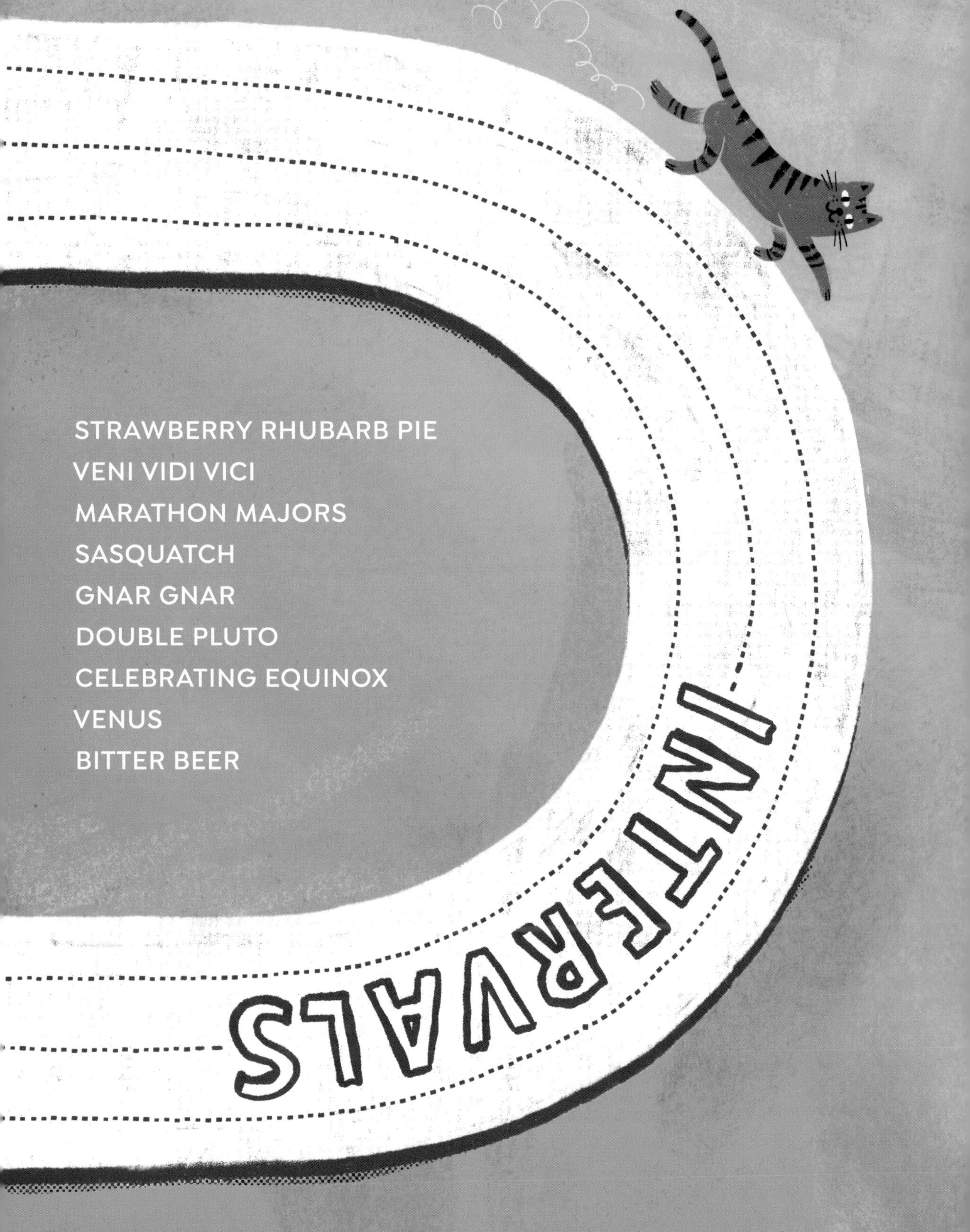

STRAWBERRY RHUBARB PIE

VENI VIDI VICI

MARATHON MAJORS

SASQUATCH

GNAR GNAR

DOUBLE PLUTO

CELEBRATING EQUINOX

VENUS

BITTER BEER

INTERVALS

$$\theta = \frac{2\pi}{\phi^2} n, \quad r = c\sqrt{n}$$

florets in the head
of a sunflower

$$\sqrt{1 + \sqrt{1 + \sqrt{1 + \ldots}}}$$

$$F = \phi^i - \phi^i$$

$$\frac{-\sqrt{5}}{2}$$

$$\sin\left(\frac{x}{2} - i \ln \phi\right) = \frac{\sqrt{5}}{2}$$

$$\frac{i}{2}$$

$$= 1 + e$$

$$\phi = \frac{1 + \sqrt{5}}{2}$$

$$\phi^{n-1} + \phi^{n-2}$$

$$\phi \approx 1.$$

$$+ \frac{1}{1 + \frac{1}{e}}$$

$$e = \frac{1}{1 + \frac{1}{1 +}}$$

0 1 1 2 3 5 8 13 21

$$\phi \approx 1.618$$

Fibonacci

0 1 1 2 3 5 8 13 21 34...

DISTANCES: 800 strides, 400, 400, 800, 1200, 2000, 3200

- -

LUNG BURN: 🔥 🔥 🔥

Italian mathematician Leonardo of Pisa is often credited with introducing the world, in his 1202 book, to the Fibonacci sequence. Of course, as you surely remember from history, the sequence had largely been figured out by Indian mathematician Pingala 1,400 years earlier in a work enumerating Sanskrit poetry patterns. The Fibonacci sequence, 1-1-2-3-5-8, turns up all the time in mathematics as well as in nature. A pine cone's bracts, the fruit sprouts of a pineapple, the seed pattern in a sunflower all follow the beautifully spiraling numerical sequence.

For today's loops around the track, we'll spiral a little beauty for ourselves. Each number in the Fibonacci sequence equals the number of laps in the interval. For intervals longer than a single lap, we'll spiral into the outer lanes of the track. If you're interested in developing more Fibonaccian workouts, feel free to subscribe to *The Fibonacci Quarterly*.

HOW TO RUN IT

Begin with 800m of strides (these don't count toward your Fibonacci, only your warmup). For each interval after that, start in lane 1 and move out a lane for every lap. The Fibonacci ideal is to maintain the same lap time, regardless of lane number. Run the shorter intervals at your 5k pace. For the longer intervals, try running the first lap in lane 1 at your 10k pace. From there, you'll need to gradually increase the pace to maintain lap times as you spiral to the outer lanes.

REST INTERVAL

60-second active rest between intervals

HERE'S WHERE IT HURTS

This workout progressively builds in intensity, especially when you get to the final three intervals. The inventor of the 8-lane track will be thoroughly cursed throughout the last half of your 3200. It will not feel beautiful.

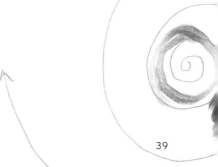

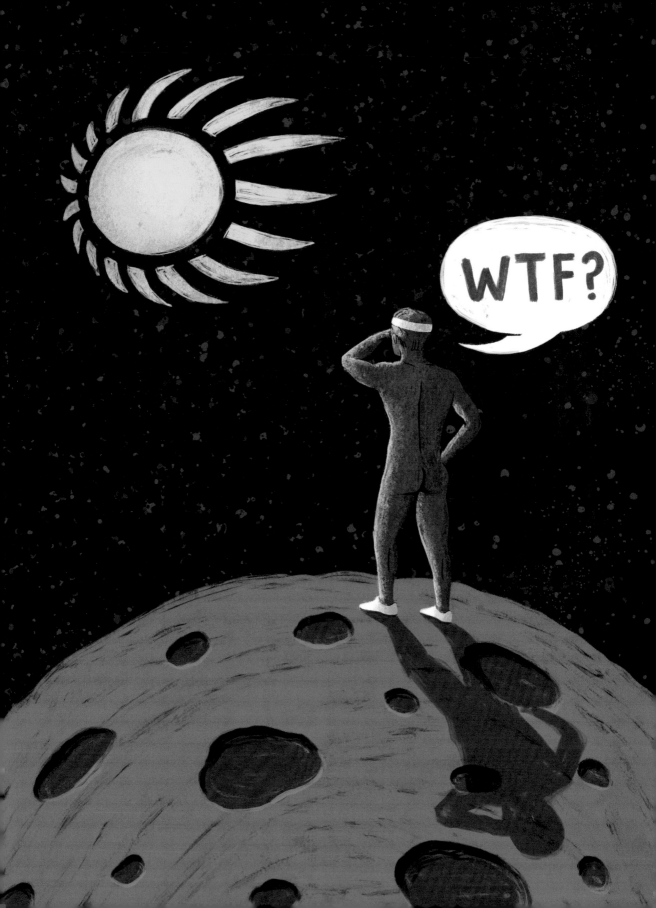

Vacation to Mercury

DISTANCES: 4 x 500, 1000, 4 x 500, 1000, 4 x 500

- -

LUNG BURN:

Due to orbit times around the Sun and Earth's own rotational speed, planets can occasionally appear to go into what's called retrograde orbit, meaning if you're paying close attention, they look as though they unexpectedly move in the opposite direction. (It's just an optical illusion, something you may be familiar with given your appetite for track intervals.)

Mercury retrogrades, but we can't see it because the Sun obscures the illusion. But if you, intrepid runner, were to holiday on the surface of Mercury, you'd actually get to see the Sun go into retrograde. Why? Sometimes Mercury's orbital speed exceeds its rotational velocity, and at those times the Sun would appear to rise, reverse course, and set where it just came up, all in the same day. This would, of course, be the highlight of your trip. The word retrograde, by the way, comes from the Latin *retrogradus*, which means backward step. Which is all a long way of getting to the astro trivia we plan to employ for this workout.

HOW TO RUN IT

Run the 500s at your 5k pace. Run the 1000s at your 10k pace. Jog the rests retrogradely, or backward, to your starting line.

REST INTERVAL

After each 500, slowly jog backward 100m; 45-second active rest after the 1000s

HERE'S WHERE IT HURTS

Sure there are times during this workout when you'll convince yourself the discomfort is just not worth whatever theoretical gain. But the true hurt comes from the humiliation of running backward when you're utterly gassed.

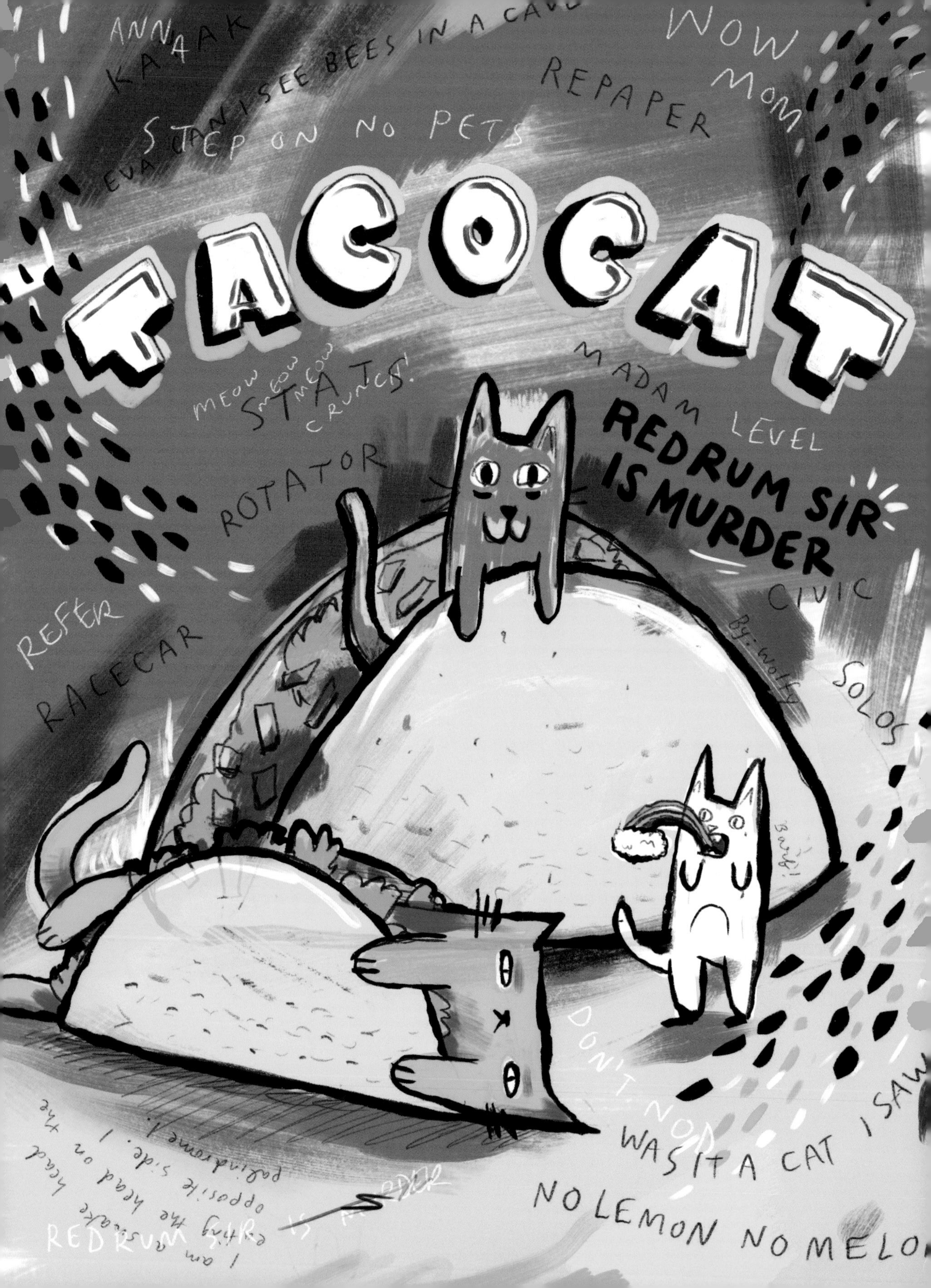

ANNA AK

KA

EVA STAN I SEE BEES IN A CAV

STEP ON NO PETS

REPAPER

WOW
MOM

TACOCAT

meow meow STATS!
SMEOW CRUNCH!

MADAM LEVEL

REDRUM SIR
IS MURDER

ROTATOR

REFER

RACECAR

CIVIC

By: wolf

SOLOS

Bark!

DON'T NOD

WAS IT A CAT I SAW

NO LEMON NO MELO

REDRUM SIR IS MURDER

I am awake head on the
head on the opposite side.
pgfindsome!

Palindrome

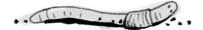

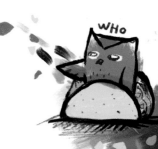

DISTANCES: 800, 1200, 1200, 800, 2000, 1600

- -

LUNG BURN: 🔥🔥🔥🔥

As a lover of running circles around a track, you're already an honorary palindrome aficionado. Congratulations! Palindromes, of course, are words, sentences, or phrases spelled exactly the same way forward as backward. *Radar*, *kayak*, *toot*, and *noon* are examples of common one-word palindromes.

Sentence palindromes often careen into Dada land: *Step on no pets* or *Eva, can I stab bats in a cave?* For today's workout, we'll take full advantage of *Mr Owl ate my metal worm*. Near the end, your oxygen-starved mind will decide *suffer* is definitely a palindrome.

HOW TO RUN IT

Each letter in Mr Owl's palindrome represents a lap, each word equals an interval, and the spaces between the words are the rest. So *Mr* is a 2-lap interval, while *Owl* is a 3-lap interval. Run the consonant laps at your 10k pace and the vowel laps a bit faster than your 5k pace. We'll let you decide how to categorize the *y* in *my*. Vowel or not?

REST INTERVAL

60-second active rest between intervals

HERE'S WHERE IT HURTS

Things are likely a mess already, but when you hit the *a* during the *metal* interval, things get appropriately hard—as in pop-a-lung hard. You may wish Mr Owl had instead decided to eat a worm with fewer letters and vowels. But that wouldn't be a palindrome, would it?

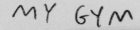

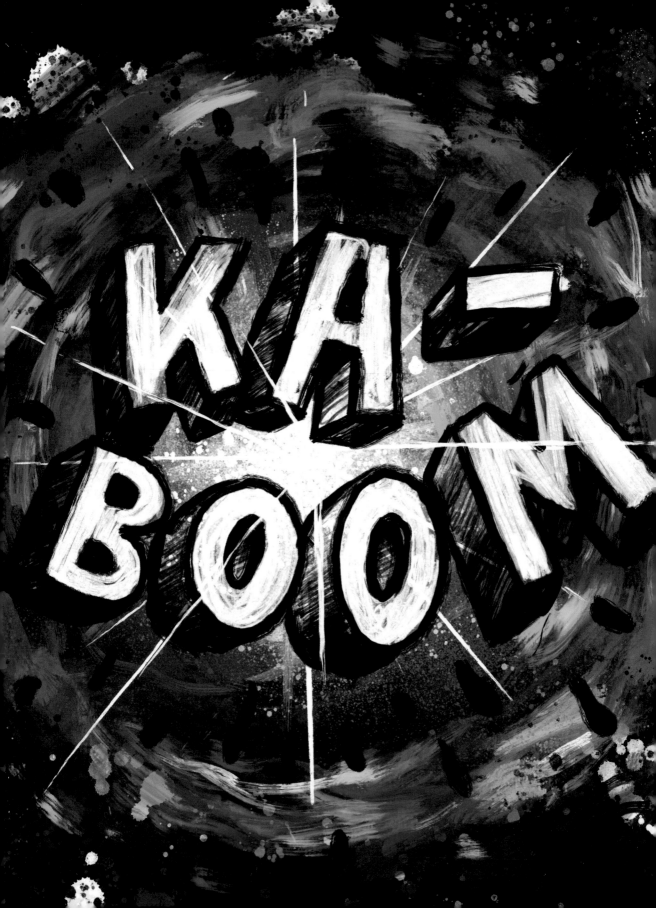

Betelgeuse

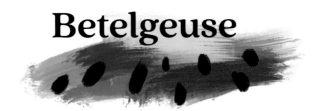

DISTANCES: 1600, 1200, 800, 400, 800, 3200

- -

LUNG BURN: 🔥 🔥

Our sun has been around for 4.6 billion years, and astronomers tell us it has 4 billion good years left, give or take. At that time, it will likely bloat out to become a red giant. Not all stars live so long, and they don't all slowly swell when they die. Some bigger stars have short lives and dramatic endings. Betelgeuse, the huge reddish star that marks Orion's shoulder and one of the brightest in the night sky, has only existed for 8 million years. That means some of our earliest, possibly bipedal running ancestors never even saw it.

Betelgeuse has recently dimmed, and some astronomers believe it could be ready to explode into a supernova. That's what happens when an enormous star runs out of juice then contracts until its tightly squeezed matter suddenly explodes. At about 600 light years from Earth, Betelgeuse may have already blown up and we just haven't seen it yet. But you have a workout calendar based on Earth time, not space time. So while Betelgeuse may have already exploded, your intervals have yet to be run. Out to the track!

HOW TO RUN IT

As your star slowly contracts, run at your 5k pace for the 1600 and the 1200. The dark matter in your brain squeezes tightly as you run the 800s and the 400 faster than your 5k pace. Your star explodes during the 3200: Run it at your 10k pace.

REST INTERVAL

60-second active rest between intervals

HERE'S WHERE IT HURTS

The whole point of this workout is to explode after 3 miles of pretty hard running. So it's during your final 2-mile interval where things get rough. The question is, are you going to bloat like a red giant, implode into a black hole, or explode in a beautiful supernova?

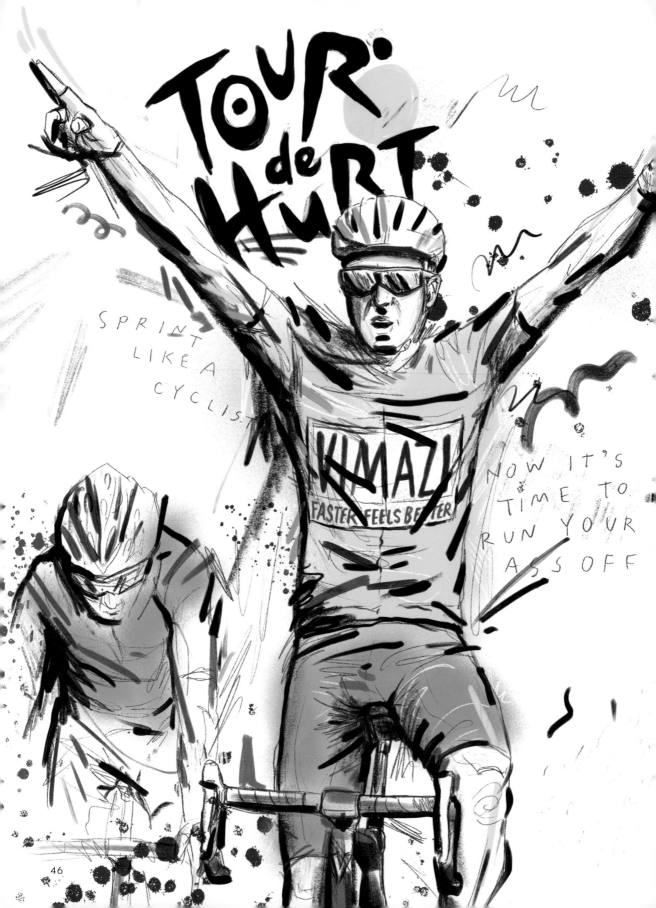

Tour de Hurt

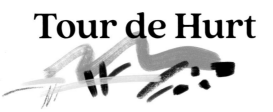

DISTANCES: 7 x 4 minutes

- -

LUNG BURN: 🔥🔥🔥🔥

There's more than one winner of the Tour de France each summer. Yes, one guy wins the General Classification, meaning he rode the three-week course in less time than everyone else. But there's also a King of the Mountains winner, a Best Young Rider winner, and a Points (Best Sprinter) winner. For that last classification, riders can earn points by winning intermediate sprints (sometimes called *primes*) that take place multiple times during each day's race. A rider can also accumulate points by winning the day's race. To win this classification, all you need to do is win more sprint points than anyone else. Cake!

You can probably see where this is going. Inspired by the race-within-a-race concept, we're going to run some sprints within intervals. Note: This is the only workout that uses time rather than set distances for the intervals.

HOW TO RUN IT
Start running at your 10k pace. At the 600m mark, run your intermediate sprint for 200m, then keep running hard until you hit 4 minutes. Here's the gut punch: For each successive interval, try to run a little farther than you ran the one before.

REST INTERVAL
90-second active rest between intervals

HERE'S WHERE IT HURTS
If you think this is an easy workout, then you didn't play fair during the first four intervals. It should start out tough and finish in a phlegmy pool that used to be called your muscles.

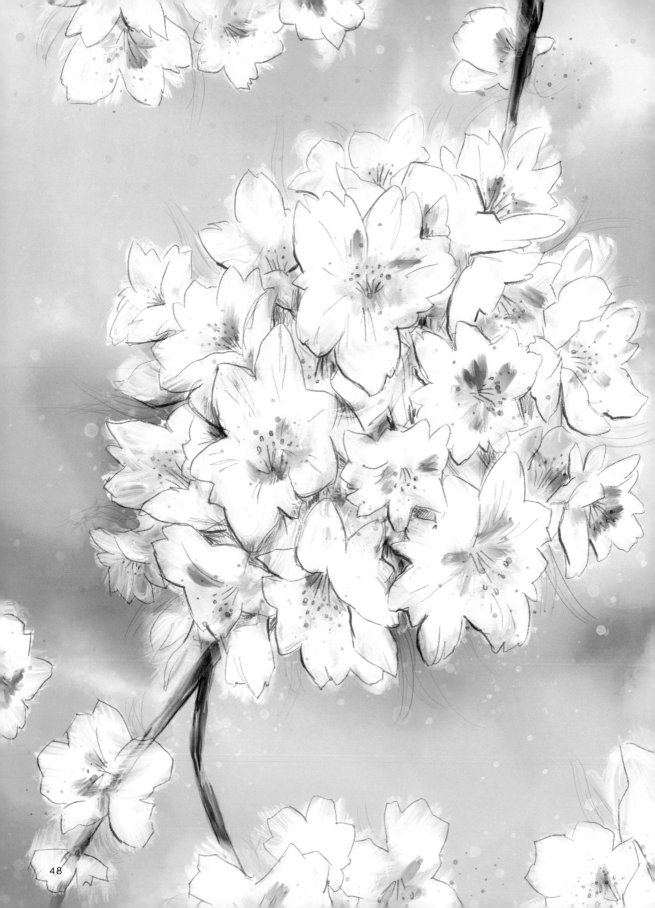

Cherry Blossoms

DISTANCES: 2 x (1600, 4 x 400, 800, 200)

- -

LUNG BURN: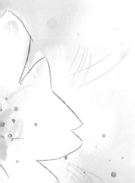

The annual blooming of the cherry blossoms is one of the most beautiful sights in Portland, Oregon. (And there are many!) When the sun finally comes out in March or April after a long, wet winter—to fanfare all around, especially from runners—the cherry trees blossom out. Sap surges into the branches, buds form, and flowers open. But by early May the blossoms have fallen to the ground, the wind blows them away, and we all have to wait another year.

One of the best places to check out the pink blossoms also happens to be a great place to run. Tom McCall Waterfront Park in downtown Portland, right along the Willamette River, sports a few miles of scenic, in-city running, with connections to trails beyond. The lovely springtime rhythm of Portland's cherry blossoms gives us the natural template for this workout.

HOW TO RUN IT

Run the 1600s (sap surging) and 800s (blossoms falling) at your 10k pace. Run the 400s (blossoms blooming) slightly faster than your 5k pace. Sprint the 200s (a brisk wind). Finish each interval with your arms up, enthralled and gratified by the beauty of the world.

REST INTERVAL

60-second active rest after the 1600s;
30-second active rest between the 400s;
45-second active rest on either side of the 800s;
2-minute active rest between sets

HERE'S WHERE IT HURTS

Coming after a 1600 and with only 30 seconds of rest between them, it doesn't take long before the 400s take a two-by-four to your legs. If you can actually sprint the 200 at the end of the second set, you may need to have a conversation with yourself about your commitment level.

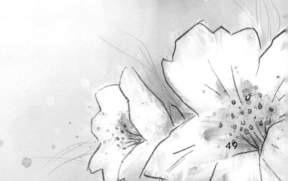

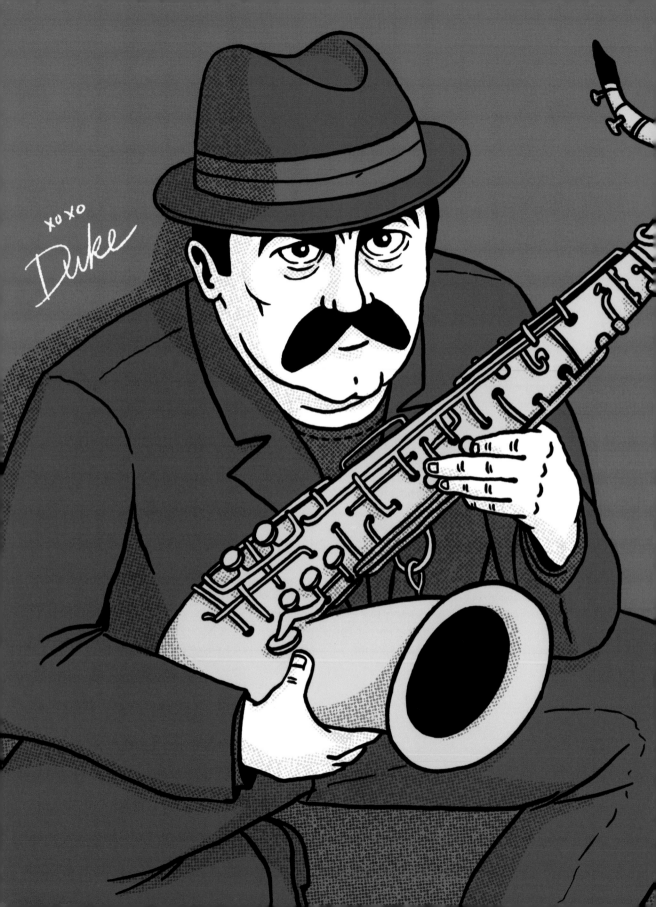

Run Your Scales

It's about to get all warm up in my jazz.

DISTANCES: 1200, 1600, 2000, 1600, 1200, 400

- -

LUNG BURN: 🔥 🔥 🔥 🔥

If you ever took lessons and learned how to play an instrument, you likely know a little about reading music. The treble clef, so called when the G clef is located on the second line from the bottom of the staff, is often where beginning musicians start practicing scales. After mastering a few basics, they add rhythm and intensity levels to their practice. In this workout, like any conscientious music student, we'll run our scales and play with intensities.

Some instruments, like the piano, incorporate both bass and treble clefs, but many learn-how-to-play-and-breathe-at-the-same-time wind instruments rely solely on the higher treble clef notes. Think bagpipe, clarinet, flute, most horns, and saxophone. Breathing, we'll helpfully point out, is necessary for playing music and running intervals. After this particular set of ovals, you may wish you'd done a lot more breathing practice.

HOW TO RUN IT

Run these intervals at your 10k pace with the following exceptions: Run slightly faster than your 5k pace on lap 1 of the first interval, lap 2 of the second, lap 3 of the third, lap 4 of the fourth, and lap 2 of the fifth. Run the final 400 much faster than your 5k pace. That's how you play with intensities.

REST INTERVAL

60-second active rest between intervals

HERE'S WHERE IT HURTS

It'll be freaking hard to hit those high notes on the second and third laps of your fifth interval. And if you can roll into a good, high-intensity final 400, you're performing better than most. But most likely you're going to feel like you've blown your sax's octave vent by the time this is all over.

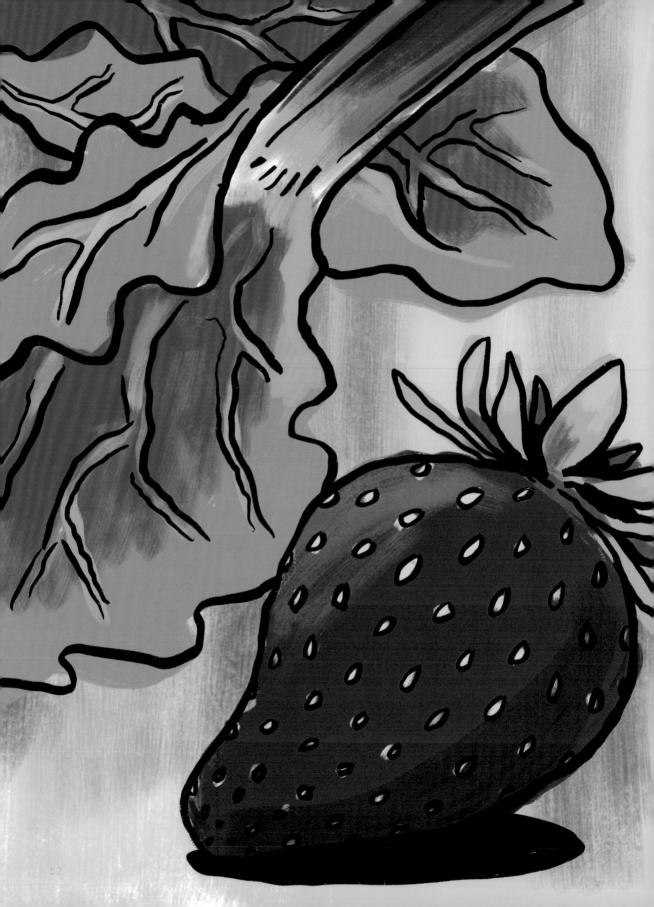

Strawberry Rhubarb Pie

DISTANCES: 3 x 1200, 8 x 300, 5 x 400

- -

LUNG BURN: 🔥🔥🔥🔥

Fruit pies are awesome. Since they contain each of the three primary food groups that power any healthy runner—pastry, fruit, and sugar—fruit pies may be the perfect food. Our favorite is strawberry rhubarb. We're pretty sure we have an entire brain lobe devoted to it, with one zone processing sweet, juicy strawberries while another cycles on tart, zingy rhubarb. One of life's great disappointments is that we can't enter strawberry rhubarb pie into the training logs.

We can, however, bake up a workout. Sugary juices ensure a bottom crust that's satisfyingly chewy and sweet, thus the 1200s. The insides—with strawberries, rhubarb, plus a little salt, flour, and butter—have the otherworldly juicy-sweet tang reminiscent of a bunch of 300s. The lattice crust, sign of a dedicated 400m connoisseur, comes out light and crisp. As this is one of the year's first fresh fruit pies, you might sample this workout in late spring or early summer.

HOW TO RUN IT

For the 1200s, run the first lap faster than your 5k pace and the remaining two laps at your 10k pace. Sprint the 300s, taking a very short break between each. The 400s should be run as progressions, so start each at your 5k pace and accelerate to a sprint by the end.

REST INTERVAL

60-second active rest between 1200s and 400s; 10-second rest between 300s

HERE'S WHERE IT HURTS

To be honest, we'd eat up those lower-crust 1200s any day of the week. But with some simple math you'll notice your sweet strawberry-rhubarb filling, the 300s, adds up to nearly 2 miles of sprinting with very little rest. Like your pie, it's the best part, and it'll hurt a lot.

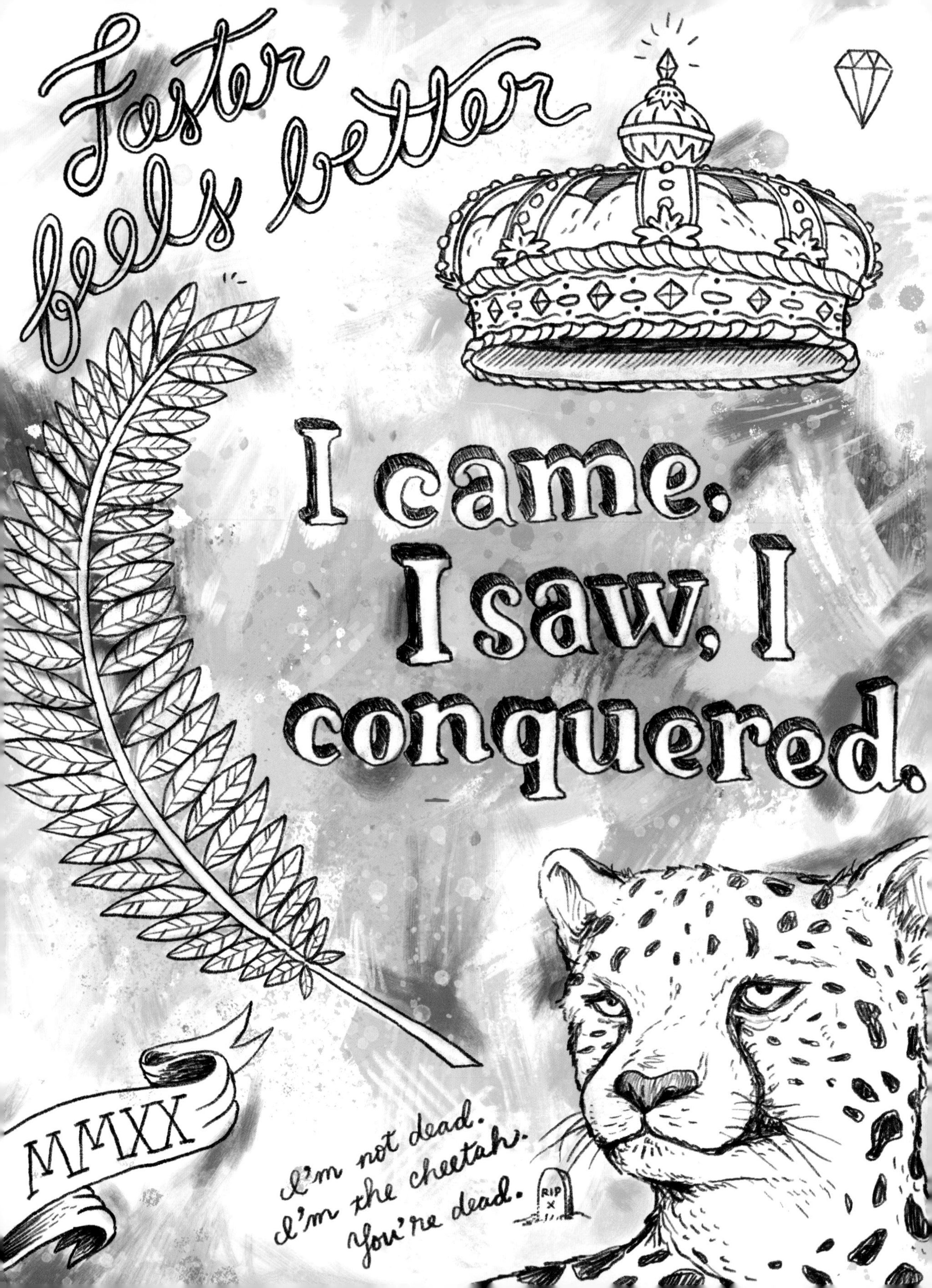
Faster feels better
I came, I saw, I conquered.
MMXX
I'm not dead.
I'm the cheetah.
You're dead.
RIP
X

Veni Vidi Vici

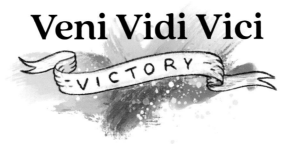

DISTANCES: 3 x (1200, 400, 700, 400)

- -

LUNG BURN: 🔥 🔥 🔥 🔥

Julius Caesar had a pretty big ego, but even in his wildest dreams he couldn't have imagined that a pithy note he sent to the Roman Senate back in 47 BC would be in such common use today. After achieving a speedy, catlike victory against Pharnaces II at the Battle of Zela, Caesar quickly scribbled "Veni, Vidi, Vici," then sent a courier on his way to deliver the message. Translated as "I came, I saw, I conquered," Caesar had, it seems, already mastered the art of writing pithy Instagram captions.

Over time, the quip has been widely used and adapted. From the Billie Holiday lyric "You came, you saw, you conquered me" to the famous *Ghostbusters* line "We came, we saw, we kicked its ass" to Madonna's song "Veni, Vidi, Vici," Caesar's words live on. The trouble here is that if you decide to run Veni, Vidi, Vici, you may not conquer. You may not even kick ass. You may, in fact, feel less like Caesar and a lot more like Pharnaces II. May luck be with you.

HOW TO RUN IT

The Vs stand for 1200, the vowels are 400, and the other consonants are assigned 700. That's how you conquer. Each of the three sets gets progressively faster. Run the Veni set at your 10k pace, the Vidi at your 5k pace, and the Vici faster than your 5k pace.

REST INTERVAL

30-second active rest between intervals; 2-minute active rest between sets

HERE'S WHERE IT HURTS

Yes, defeat in battle can be painful. But we're here to prove that even if you come, see, and conquer, it can be equally brutal. We're talking jetpack-misfire-off-a-tall-cliff-holding-an-anvil-only-to-have-a-boulder-land-on-your-head brutal. Oh, that's never happened to you before? Run your Vici set and then let's talk.

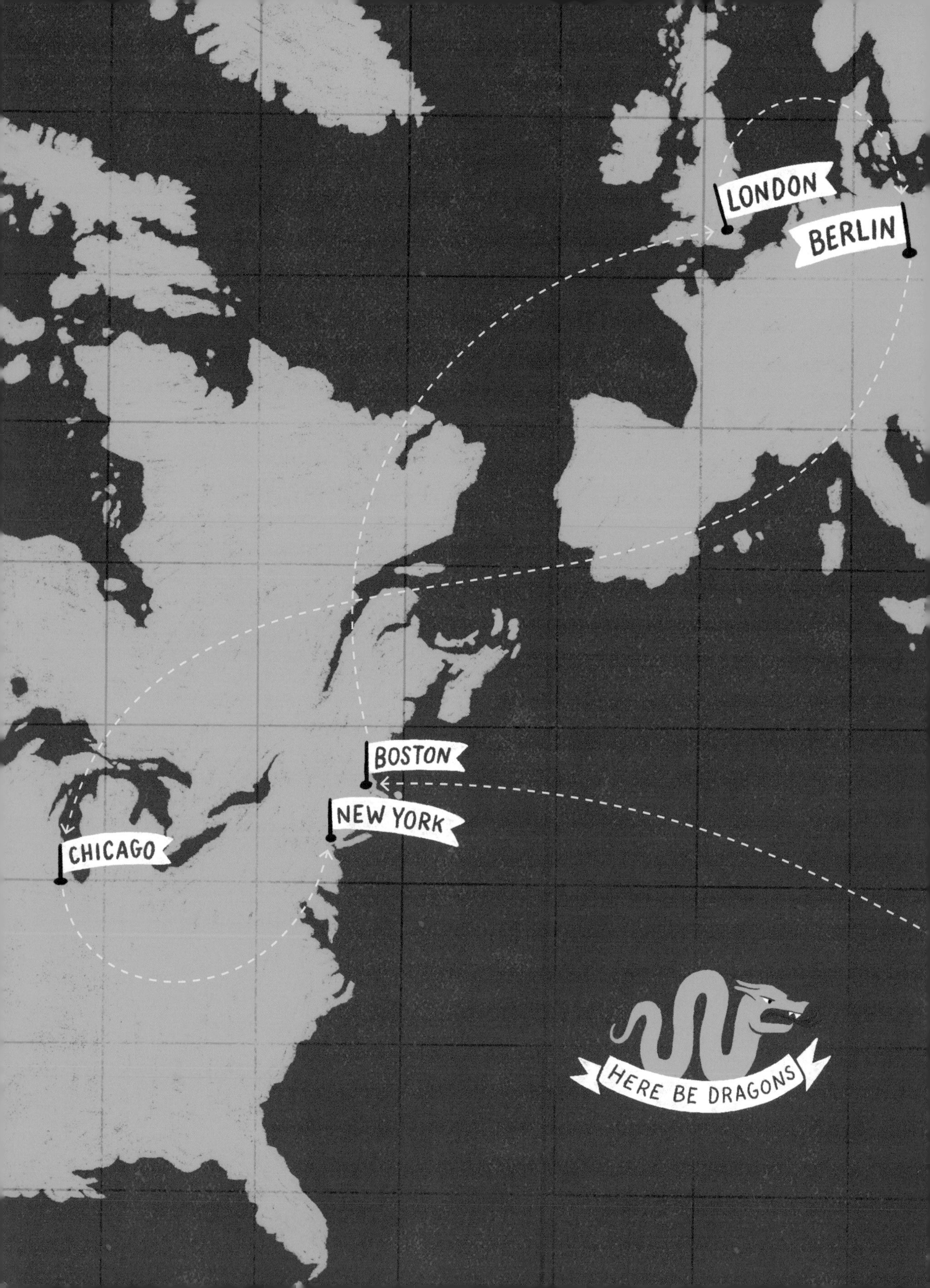
LONDON
BERLIN
BOSTON
NEW YORK
CHICAGO
HERE BE DRAGONS

Marathon Majors

DISTANCES: 800, 1200, 1200, 1200, 1600, 1600

- -

LUNG BURN: 🔥 🔥 🔥 🔥

For its legendary history, phenomenal participation, and blood-and-sweat challenge, the marathon captures the imagination more than any other distance. Just take the story (and it's likely just a story) of Philippides—who ran from Marathon to Athens in 490 BC to deliver news of military victory then promptly keeled over and died—and you'll understand why the marathon occupies more mental trophy-shelf space than, say, the 10,000 meters ever will.

About 800 marathons are held each year, but only six of them have become big, prestigious, and fast enough to be considered a World Marathon Major. Each year, in this order, runners toe the line at the Tokyo, Boston, London, Berlin, Chicago, and New York marathons. For this workout, a five-letter major city equals 2 laps, a six-letter major equals 3 laps, and a seven-letter major equals 4 laps. Running all six majors is a huge accomplishment, and now you can run them all in a single workout. Woof!

HOW TO RUN IT

These are meant to be long, hard intervals. Run them all at your 5k pace, but run the second lap of each interval slightly faster than your 5k pace.

REST INTERVAL

60-second active rest between intervals

HERE'S WHERE IT HURTS

You may get away with feeling good on your Tokyo and even Boston intervals, but once you hit London's intensity lap, it's all snot, misery, and heartache.

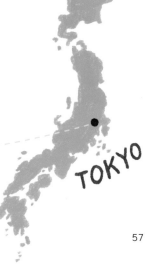

TOKYO

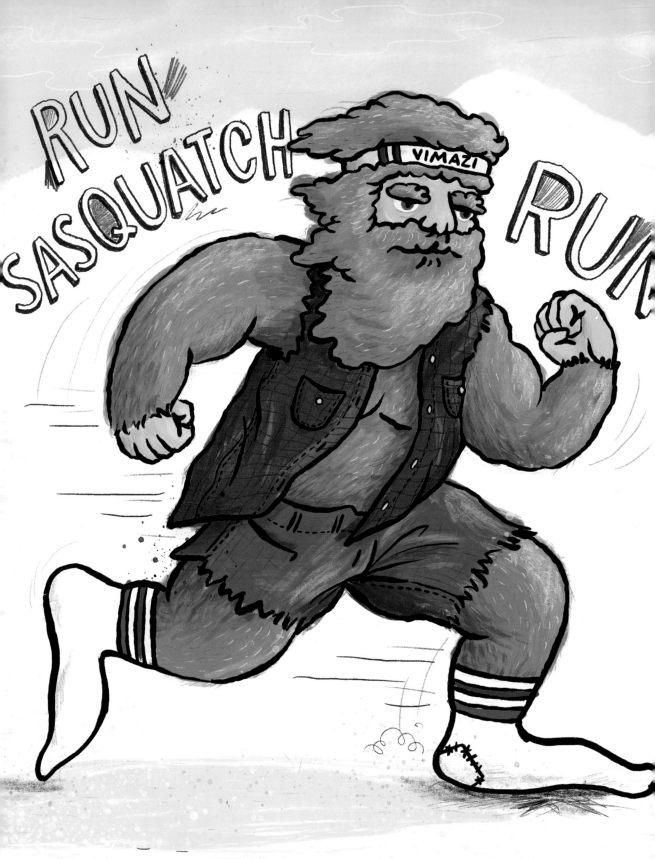

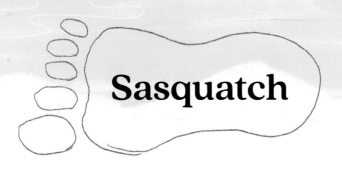

Sasquatch

DISTANCES: 4000, 5 x 800

- -

LUNG BURN: 🔥🔥

Being from the Pacific Northwest, we share our home region with Sasquatch, also known as Bigfoot, cousin to the Himalayan yeti. Okay, okay. We can sense the dismissal in your breath, the reflexive tensing of your opposable thumb, the revving of higher logic in your cortex. Well, as the bumper sticker goes, *Sasquatch doesn't believe in you either.* Perhaps Sasquatch is just really expert at avoiding contact. Between 1818 and 1980, there were more than 1,000 sightings, all fleeting and most occurring in the coastal and inland mountains between British Columbia and Northern California. Could they really all be bupkis?

It seems we've gotten distracted and there needs to be a workout here somewhere, so let's find one. As you'd imagine, at nearly 7 feet tall, Sasquatch has the feet of a behemoth. They're rumored to be 24 inches long and 8 inches wide, with five fist-sized toes. So, in honor of our region's mascot incognito, we'll run one big foot and five big toes. (We'll leave the number-of-toes debate for another day.)

HOW TO RUN IT

Run the 4000 at your 10k pace. While running, change lanes each lap to avoid detection. Here's your lane sequencing: 1-2-3-4-3-2-1-2-3-4. For the toe intervals, run the 800s as progressions, starting with your 10k pace and gradually accelerating to faster than your 5k pace by the end.

REST INTERVAL

2-minute active rest after the 4000;
60-second active rest between the 800s

HERE'S WHERE IT HURTS

The first 2.5 miles are pretty tough because you'll be running at your 10k race pace for nearly half a 10k, which takes a physical and mental toll on the track. But if you really push the 800s, that's where you'll feel small and insignificant. Rabbit will be unimpressed.

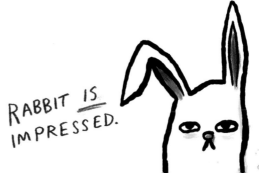

RABBIT IS IMPRESSED.

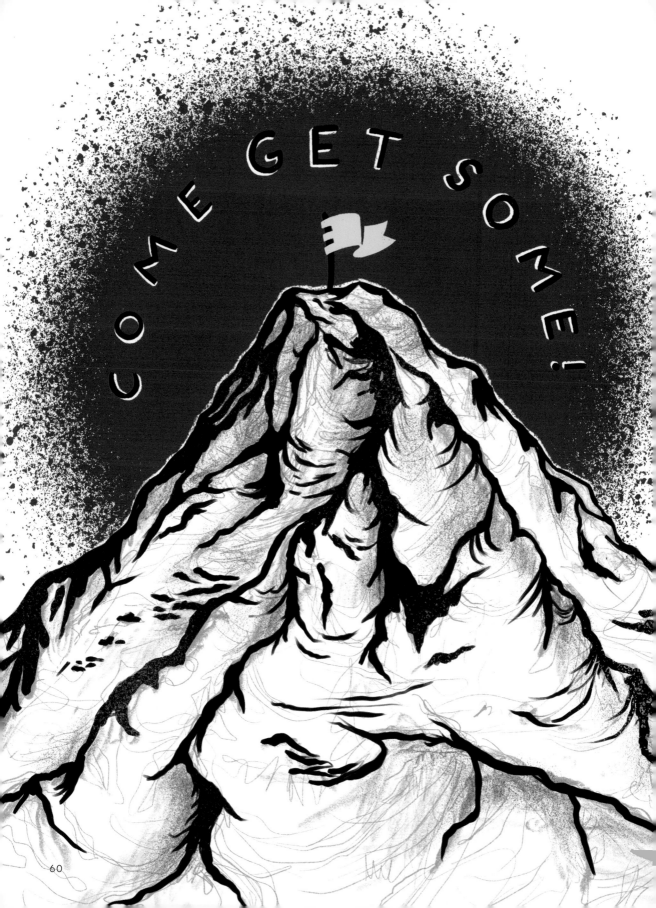

Gnar Gnar

DISTANCES: 2 × (1200, 1200, 400, 1200)

- -

LUNG BURN:

A gnashing of teeth? A mocking taunt? A steeper-than-shit trail? As it turns out, all three apply to the Gnar Gnar trail race, which is held every summer at Skibowl on the stunning southern flank of Mount Hood in Government Camp, Oregon. Ho hum, just another one of the Pacific Northwest's 11,000-foot-plus snowcapped volcanoes.

The course follows the Sunrise and Summit Trails, both of which sound like delightful jaunts through beautiful wildflower meadows. That may be, but all you'll remember is the Gnar Gnar Trail, which charges straight up the mountain at an ungodly clip. Up! It's the polar opposite of a no-turns tuck downhill during the ski season. Too bad for you it's summer. If you've ever run this race, *Gnar Gnar* may already be painfully tattooed into your memory, so you should have an easier time remembering how this workout proceeds.

HOW TO RUN IT

To run a Gnar, the consonants stand for 1200s and the vowel for 400. Start each 1200 in lane 3 and run a bit faster than your 10k pace. As you complete each lap, move in a lane and pick up the pace. By the third lap you should be running at your 5k pace. Run the 400 slightly faster than your 5k pace. When you've completed one Gnar, take a short break then start the second.

REST INTERVAL

45-second active rest between intervals; 2-minute active rest between sets

HERE'S WHERE IT HURTS

At some point during your second Gnar it'll begin to feel like the track has a steep hill in it. Time to pick up the pace.

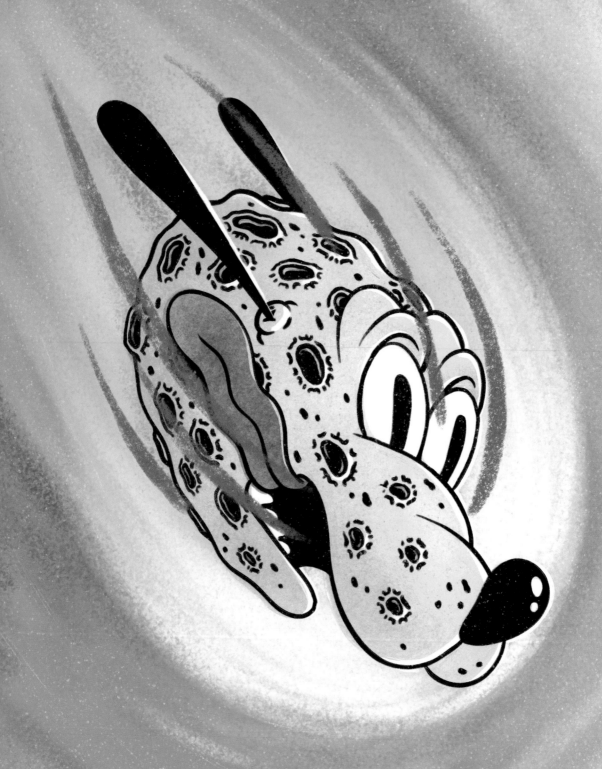

Double Pluto

DISTANCES: 2 x 2000, 2 x 900, 2 x 200, 2 x 600, 2 x 500

- -

LUNG BURN: 🔥 🔥 🔥 🔥

Let's play number association with Pluto. Ready? Pluto counted as the 9th planet until 2006, when it was demoted to dwarf planet or, technically, a spheroidal Kuiper Belt Object (KBO). So far, five rocky chunks have earned dwarf planet status (moons don't count), and Pluto, it turns out, isn't even definitively the largest. Eris is about the same size. Pluto was discovered in 1930. Pluto the Pup, Disney's beloved cartoon dog, was also introduced in 1930. These days, Pluto's about 600 dog years old. (The multiply-by-7 rule is out of date, and the new way to calculate dog age is, well, complicated.) Finally, Pluto the KBO has an orbital period of 248 years. Facts memorized?

This workout uses the year 1930 (rounded up to 2000m) for the first set, the 9th planet (900m) for the second set, a 248-year orbit (200m) for the third set, Pluto the Pup's age (600m) for the fourth, and five dwarf planets (500m) for the final set. Since we're running two of each, this is actually a Double Pluto.

HOW TO RUN IT

For the 2000s, run the first and last laps faster than your 5k pace and the middle laps a bit faster than your 10k pace. Run the 900s and 600s faster than your 5k pace. Run the 200s and 500s quite a bit faster than your 5k pace.

REST INTERVAL

60-second active rest between intervals and sets

HERE'S WHERE IT HURTS

Beware of a slowing orbit on your 600s and a wide-eyed, tongue-slobbery re-entry flameout on the 500s.

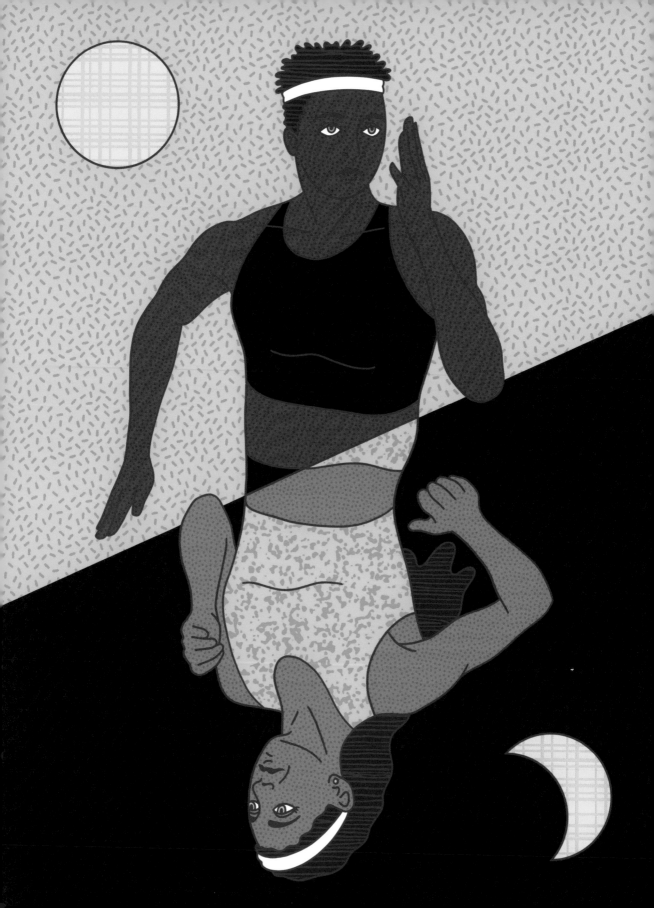

Celebrating Equinox

DISTANCES: 2 x (2400, 4 x 400)

- -

LUNG BURN:

Back in ancient times, some observant runner realized there were two days a year when night and day were of equal length. One of those days, she knew, meant six lovely months of dry sunny running ahead while the other day signified six long months of slogging along in the dark.

At some point those days were named *equinox*, which literally means equal night. And they, of course, mark the first day of spring (around March 20) or the first day of autumn (around September 22). On those two days, night and day are more or less the same duration all over the world: 12 hours of daylight, 12 hours of night. Probably the best way to celebrate is with a really, really hard workout.

HOW TO RUN IT

As you know and will likely come to regret, *autumn* has six letters. So, we'll run a 6-lap 2400 to start each set. Run the vowels somewhat faster than your 10k pace; run the consonants a bit faster than your 5k pace. All the 400s should be run much faster than your 5k pace. And since there's a spring equinox and a fall equinox, we run two sets.

REST INTERVAL

2-minute active rest after the 2400s;
30-second active rest between the 400s

HERE'S WHERE IT HURTS

At some point during your second set, in an oxygen-starved haze, your brain may try to spell autumn without the m. Nope, it's six letters and ends in two consonants, which means you'll be running the last six laps all faster than 5k pace with little rest. And you used to think celebrating equinox was a good thing.

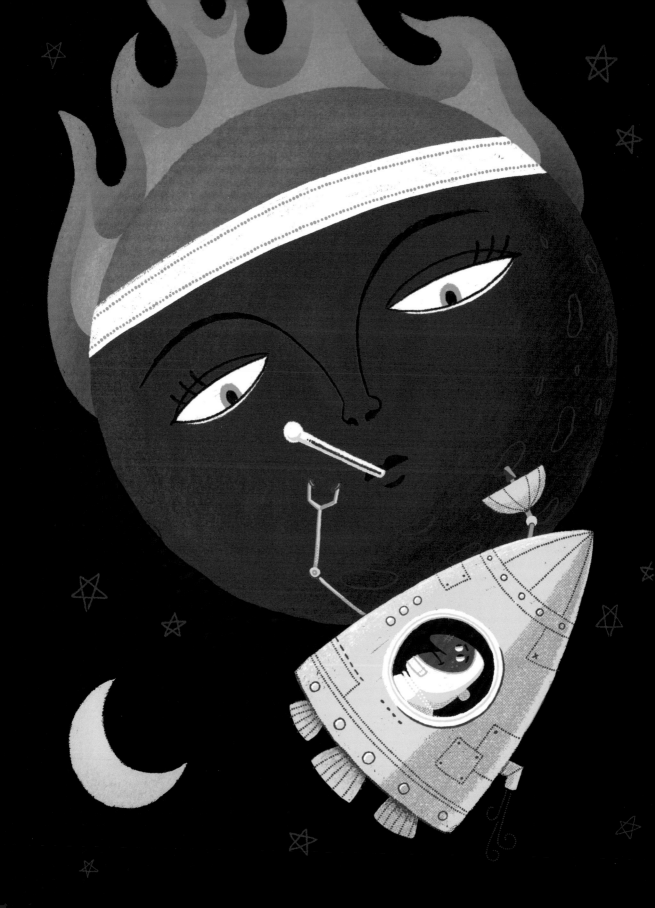

Venus

DISTANCES: 800, 2000, 800, 3200, 800, 400

- -

LUNG BURN:

Most people think Venus is Earth's closest neighbor. That distinction, however, goes to Mercury, so long as you measure using the point-circle method, which ultimately depends on whether you prefer your definitions to be of the common-sense or metaphysical variety. In any event, Venus and Earth have a few things in common: rocky cores, similar sizing, same spatial neighborhood. That's where the similarities end. Venus is insanely hot, around 863° F, due to a runaway greenhouse effect (coming to an Earth near you!), and its air pressure is 92 times ours. Venus has a synodic period of 584 days as viewed from Earth. Further, Venus has an orbital period of 224 days and a rotation period of 243 days, meaning its day is longer than its year. So birthday cakes should arrive more than once per day.

But what's the greater meaning? The three types of orbital and rotational periods mean three 800s. Duh! The 800° forecast calls for 8 laps, thus a 3200. The synodic period of 584 days gives us our 5-lap 2000, and the 1:1 size ratio means one final lap at the end. Clear as the Venusian sky!

HOW TO RUN IT
While interplanetary comparisons and celestial relationships can get complex, this workout is actually quite straightforward. Run the 800s and 400 slightly faster than your 5k pace. Run the 2000 right at your 5k pace. Run the 3200 at your 10k pace.

REST INTERVAL
60-second active rest between each interval

HERE'S WHERE IT HURTS
Kind of a coin flip here between the fast 2000 and the third 800. The synodic period of hurt is short for both.

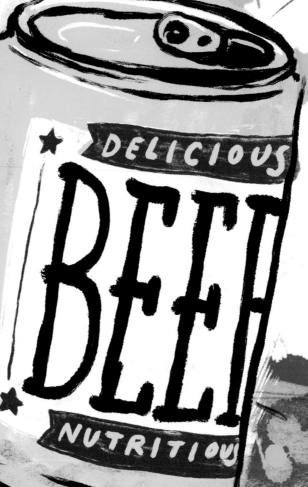

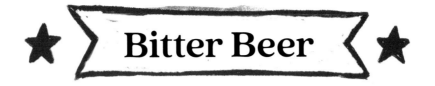

Bitter Beer

DISTANCES: 5 x 100, 5 X 200, 5 X 300, 5 x 400, 3 x 500, 3 x 600

LUNG BURN: 🔥 🔥

Beer is awesome and something many runners love. Extreme fondness can result in events like the Beer Mile, a race where you chug a 12-ouncer to start each lap.

Beer connoisseurs have lots of other ways to express and debate their passion, one being International Bitterness Units (IBUs). Beer contains isohumulone, an acid in hops, and IBUs measure the parts per million of isohumulone in a particular beer. Higher readings theoretically mean greater bitterness, but it really all depends on the recipe and how it strikes your taste buds on a given night. Here are the approximate IBUs typically found in these beers: wheat (10), lager (20), porter (30), pale ale (40), stout (50), IPA (60). Yes, we know there are credible objections to this IBU level for IPAs. If you object, feel free to increase the distance of your IPA intervals to your particular know-it-all level. Two notes: First, interval distances equal IBU levels times 10. Second, the puke penalty is a second IPA set.

HOW TO RUN IT

Run the 100s and 200s faster than your 5k pace. Run the 300s and 400s at your 5k pace. Run the 500s and 600s somewhat faster than your 10k pace.

REST INTERVAL

10-second pause between each interval; 60-second active rest between sets

HERE'S WHERE IT HURTS

Compared with many of the other workouts in this book, Bitter Beer has a mellower IBU rating and splatters less pain. Pair it with Vimazi Chips (see page 88), however, and you'll be nursing a three-day hangover. Even without the chips the last three 600s in this workout, all on little rest, may increase your bittering as a human.

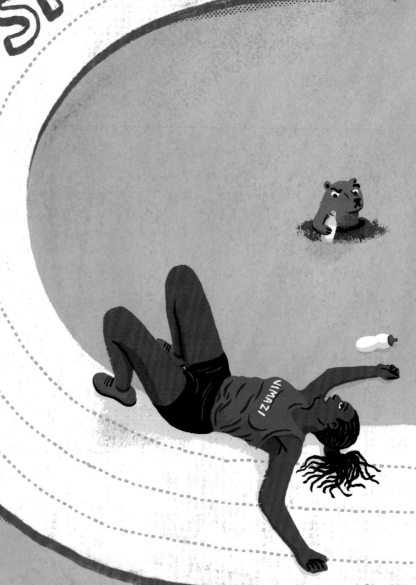

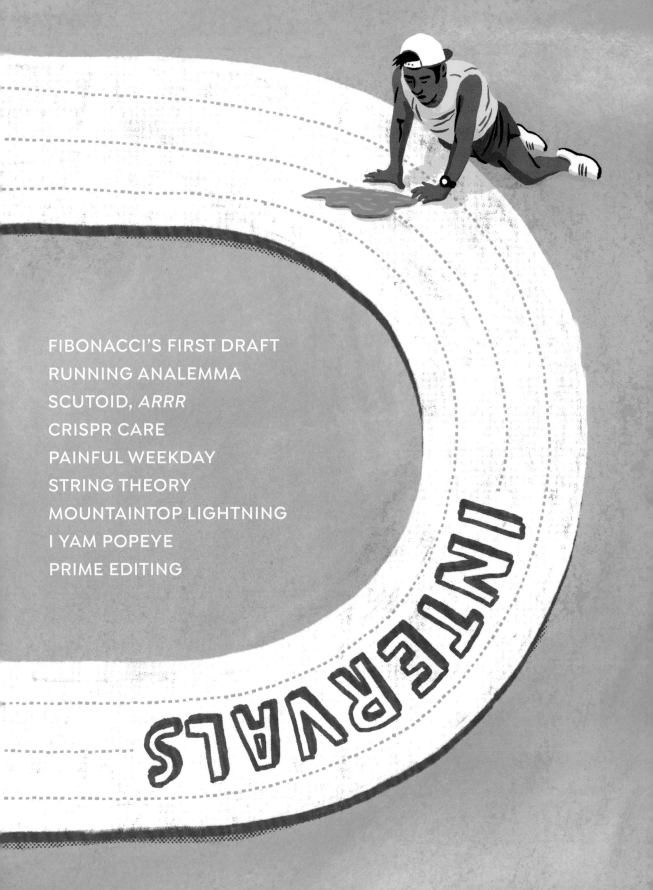

FIBONACCI'S FIRST DRAFT
RUNNING ANALEMMA
SCUTOID, *ARRR*
CRISPR CARE
PAINFUL WEEKDAY
STRING THEORY
MOUNTAINTOP LIGHTNING
I YAM POPEYE
PRIME EDITING

INTERVALS

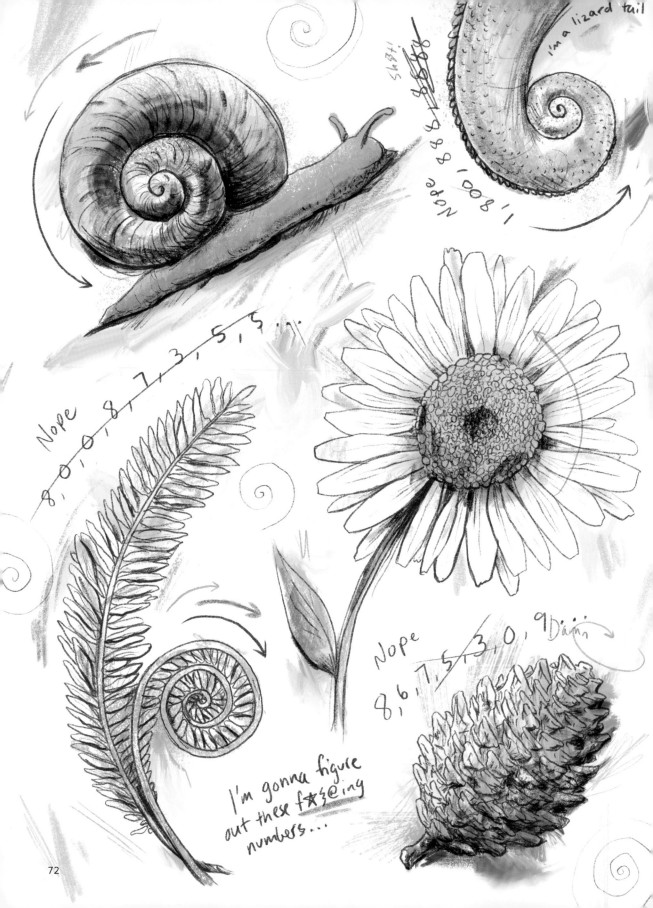

i'm a lizard tail

Slak!

Nope 1,800,888,876...

Nope 8,0,1,8,7,3,5,5...

Nope 8,6,7,5/3,0,9 Dann...

I'm gonna figure out these f*$@ing numbers...

72

Fibonacci's First Draft

2̶,̶1̶,̶4̶,̶2̶,̶5̶,̶3̶... Dammit!

DISTANCES: 5 x (200–100), 5 x (400–200), 5 x (500–300)

- -

LUNG BURN: 🔥🔥🔥🔥

Didn't we already run a Fibonacci? Yes, we did. But what many runners may not know is that Fibonacci, the 13th century Italian mathematician, didn't work out his famous sequence on the first try. It took many years, many notebooks, and many false starts before he was able to hold his 1202 book release party.

The Fibonacci sequence, deployed by nature since the dawn of time and used by mathematicians like a Swiss Army knife, is 1-1-2-3-5-8. But Fibonacci's first draft, according to our ad hoc research and back-of-a-track-meet-schedule calculations, was 2-1-4-2-5-3. This sequence, it turns out and Fibonacci ultimately realized, is utter gibberish. But we've found mathematical gibberish can sometimes be expertly repurposed into extraordinarily challenging workouts, especially when we focus on speed, multiply by five, and discard the rests. Fibonacci the runner would be proud.

HOW TO RUN IT

It will probably be helpful to think of this workout as 5 x 300, 5 x 600, and 5 x 800. For each interval, run the first part at your 10k pace then accelerate to faster than your 5k pace for the second part. Run at a fast jog to your start and do it again. So for the first interval, run a fast 200, accelerate into a very fast 100, jog 100, then immediately start the next one.

REST INTERVAL

Run at a fast jog between intervals—no walking—2-minute active rest between the three sets

HERE'S WHERE IT HURTS

While Fibonacci's sequence is naturally beautiful, his first draft creates an exceedingly hard morning at the track. You'll handle the first set just fine, but with essentially no rest, the second two sets will feel like those many years of poppycock Fibonacci notebooks. Just a reminder that there is no perfection. We're all just working on our first draft.

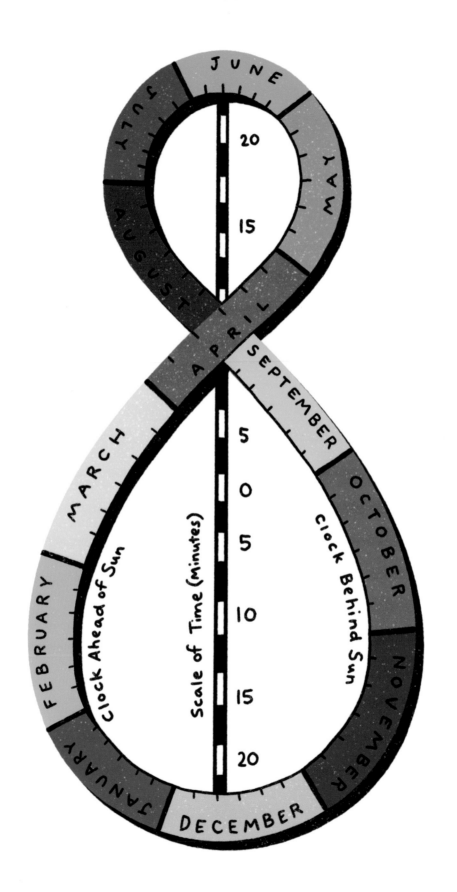

Running Analemma

DISTANCES: 4 x 800, 8 x 600

LUNG BURN:

If you live a ways away from the equator and haven't been living under a rock, you know there are a few months of the year when the Sun is overhead at noon and a few other months when it's relatively low in the sky at noon. If you photographed the Sun from your window each day at noon for an entire year, the resulting photo collage would show that the Sun traces a figure eight through the sky, not an out-and-back. The top loop (summer) is smaller than the bottom loop (winter, spring, fall), which is your penalty for not living closer to the equator.

This phenomenon is due to the Earth's tilted axis, our elliptical orbit around the Sun, and some physics, though during our daily routines most of us aren't really paying attention. The figure-eight shape of the Sun's path is called an analemma. So, we have a figure eight and we have two loops, one bigger and one smaller. Let's go.

HOW TO RUN IT

Run the first half of each interval slightly faster than your 10k pace; run the second half a bit faster than your 5k pace. For the 600s, start each new interval where the last one ended.

REST INTERVAL

45-second active rest between intervals;
2-minute active rest between sets

HERE'S WHERE IT HURTS

There will likely come a moment when you say to yourself: *Will this never end?* And while you may be able to kick it into gear during the second half of each interval, starting out each interval after such a short rest will prove the challenge, especially for the last few 600s.

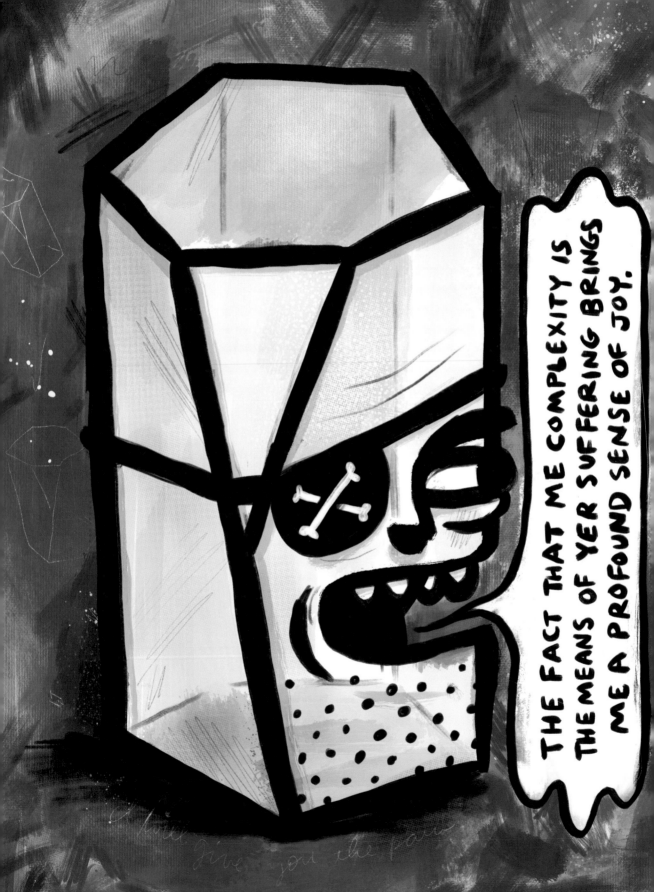

Scutoid, *ARRR*

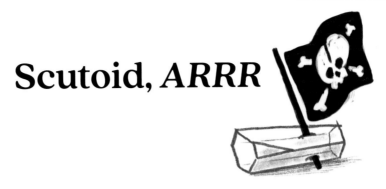

DISTANCES: 800 strides, 2 x (1 x 600, 2 x 500, 4 x 400, 1 x 300)

LUNG BURN: 🔥🔥🔥🔥

What the heck is a scutoid? And more importantly, how much will it hurt? (Answer: a lot.) A scutoid is a prismatic solid found in nature, yet only recently discovered. Its unique shape allows solids to nestle together in efficient patterns. From some angles a scutoid looks like a hexagonal prism, while from other angles it appears to be a pentagonal prism. What gives?

Turns out, one of the scutoid's prismatic panels is triangle-shaped, clipped from the hexagonal end of two adjacent trapezoidal panels. It looks a lot like a prismatoid, except that the scutoid's triangle facet doesn't extend from one end of the prism to the other. The result? Scutoids have a triangular side, four trapezoidal sides, two pentagonal sides, and a hexagonal side. And thus, a uniquely shaped workout is envisioned.

HOW TO RUN IT

These intervals are defined by scutoid facets; each edge represents 100 meters. So the hexagon equals 600m, the pentagons are 500m, the trapezoids stand for 400m, and the triangle is 300m. That's one scutoid, and you need to run two of them, plus 800m of strides to start. Run the strides and scutoid distances at your 5k pace; run the second 200m of each interval faster than your 5k pace.

REST INTERVAL

45-second active rest between intervals;
2-minute active rest between scutoids

HERE'S WHERE IT HURTS

A 5k pace seems doable, until you remember this is a 5-mile workout. *Arrr*, pain is definitely in your future. You may get through your strides and first scutoid relatively unscathed, but you'll leave guts on the track during your second scutoid, especially that second set of trapezoidal intervals.

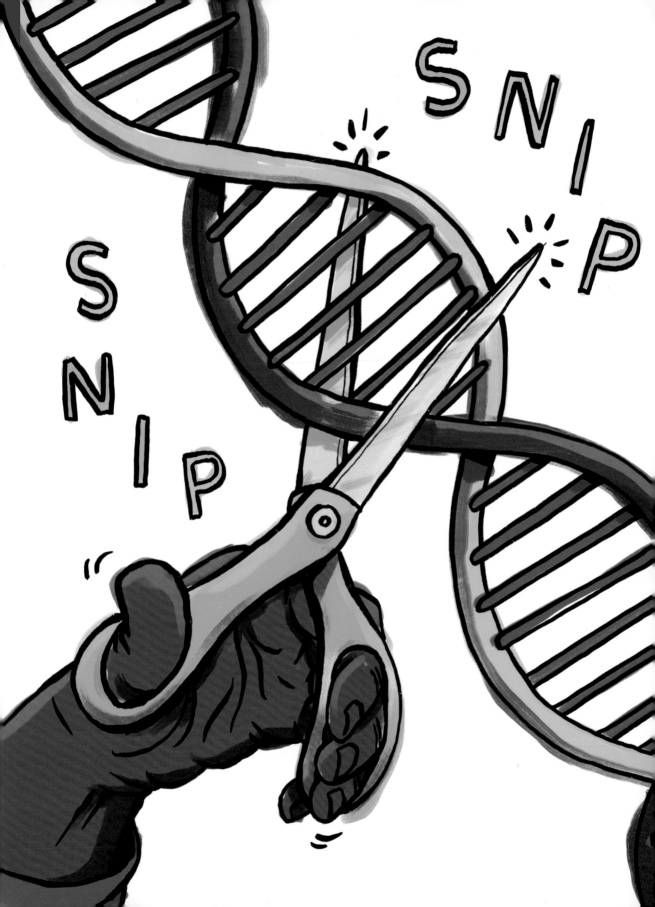

CRISPR Care

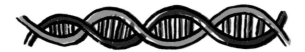

DISTANCES: 2 x (200-400-400-200, 1600, 200-400-400-200)

LUNG BURN: 🔥🔥🔥🔥🔥

A gene editing technique used in molecular biology, CRISPR stands for Clustered Regularly Interspaced Short Palindromic Repeats—which isn't exactly onomatopoetic. CRISPR associated protein 9, usually referred to as CRISPR-Cas9, is an enzyme that acts like a pair of scissors. In basic terms, the CRISPR part finds the correct location in a DNA sequence, and the Cas-9 cuts the sequence. At that point, existing genes can be removed or new genes can be added. And who among us at one time or another hasn't rued the day our parents passed us this or that lame gene? If only we could CRISPR a little self-care.

For this workout, each of the CRISPR sets, the two sets of short intervals, finds the palindromic location to cut. Since we're distance runners, a longer interval then gets inserted into our sequence. It's only then we discover: Gene-editing self-care is not for the careless. Or gutless.

HOW TO RUN IT

Run the shorter CRISPR intervals faster than your 5k pace. Run the 1600 at a steady 5k pace.

REST INTERVAL

10-second rest between the 200s and 400s; 90-second active rest on either side of the 1600s

HERE'S WHERE IT HURTS

This workout doesn't so much interspace short palindromic repeats as leave permanent scars and a lingering facial twitch. It may be the toughest workout we've included. Fast paces, short rests, and a hard mile edited into the middle will leave you a thoroughly exhausted but mentally tougher runner. Either that or a quivering pile of grape Jell-O.

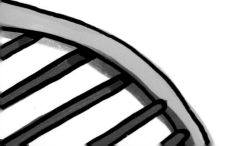

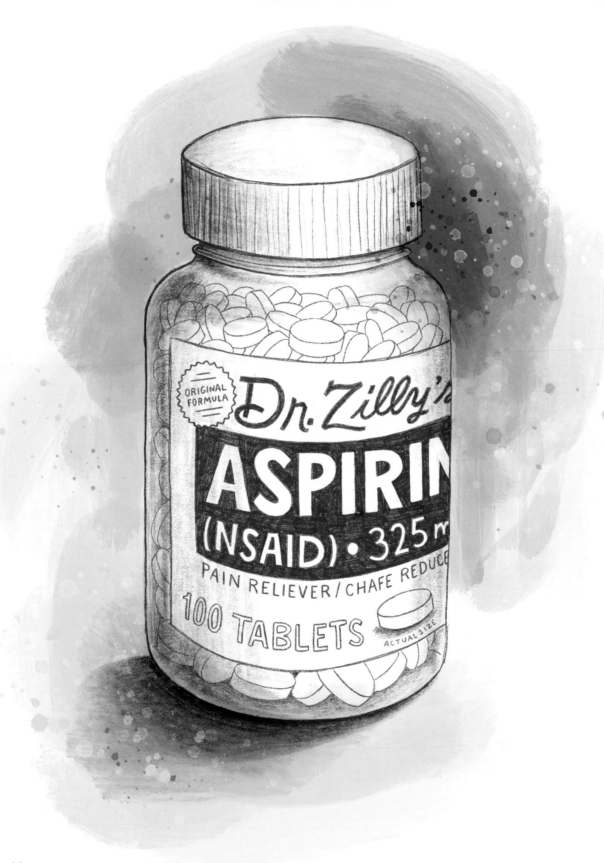

Painful Weekday

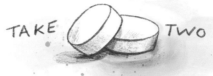

DISTANCES: 2 x 400, 2 x 400, 2 x 700, 2 x 700, 2 x 500, 2 x 600, 2 x 300, 3 x 500

- -

LUNG BURN: 🔥🔥🔥🔥🔥

Ancient Mesopotamians ingeniously used days of the week as a measurement to predict phases of the Moon. Their use of astronomy, in fact, is sometimes referred to as the first scientific revolution. With 28 days per lunar cycle (essentially a month) and four phases of the Moon per cycle, it made sense to group days into sets of seven in order to make it easier to keep track of the Moon's comings and goings (28/4 = 7 days in a week). And here we are.

As for naming the days of the week, you can cite Norse and Roman mythology plus a sprinkle of solar system: Monday for Moon, Tuesday for Mars, Wednesday for Mercury, Thursday for Jupiter, Friday for Venus, Saturday for Saturn, and Sunday is the Sun's day. If you were as smart as the Mesopotamians, you'd skip to the next workout. Since you're not, take five aspirin and read on. As the couplet distances spin outward, your orbit around the track gets longer and longer until math becomes impossible and the day of the week irrelevant.

HOW TO RUN IT

Starting with Monday, our celestial bodies proceed like this: Moon, Mars, Mercury, Jupiter, Venus, Saturn, Sun. For this workout, run 100m for each letter in the body's name. Each day is a couplet, so for Monday—Moon—run two 400s. For the 600s and shorter, run faster than your 5k pace. Run the 700s at your 5k pace. Note that your orbit changes with each couplet, so start in lane 1 for your Moon interval and move one lane out for each day. To round out the workout, break our couplet rule, and completely crush all remaining spirit: Run three 500s in lane 8.

REST INTERVAL

10-second rest between intervals;
60-second active rest between couplets

HERE'S WHERE IT HURTS

The short rest and fast pace make this one of the toughest workouts in this book. So, expect the hurt to show up early and never relent.

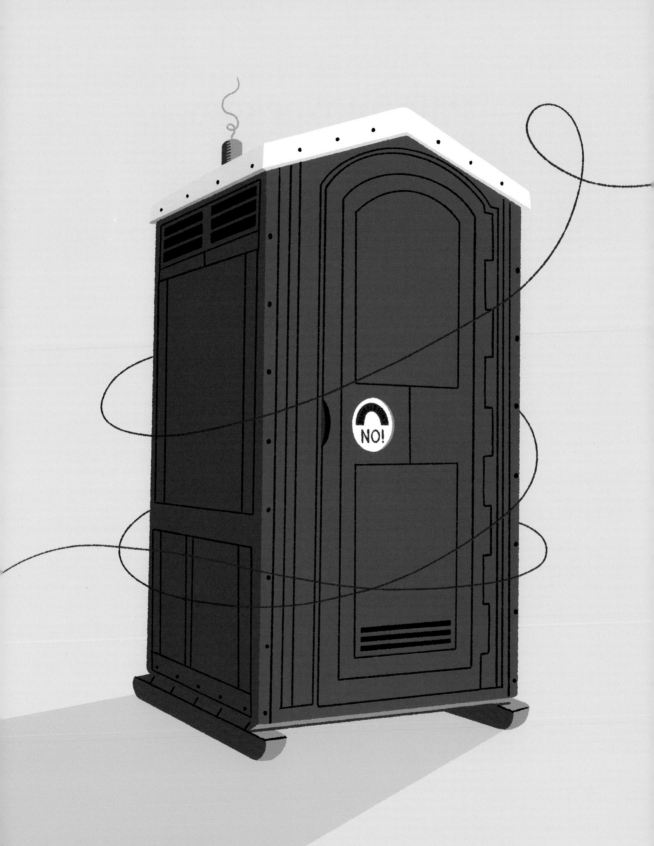

String Theory

DISTANCES: 5 x 800, 5 x 800

- -

LUNG BURN: 🔥 🔥 🔥

To be fully transparent, we've been working hard to navigate the basics of regular three-dimensional life. And we have a ways to go. That hasn't stopped know-it-all physicists from lapping us in their efforts to understand multiple other dimensions. The cosmic unfairness!

Enter superstring theory. In an effort to harmonize general relativity with quantum mechanics and, if that weren't enough, deliver the grand unified theory that explains everything, superstring theory posits a bunch of other dimensions. In this theory, tiny strings—think plucked guitar strings—vibrate at fixed frequencies. (Plus all sorts of other stuff we don't have space-time to explain.) If you run with this theory long enough, you end up in a 10-dimensional world. Let's stress test it by going out to a three-dimensional track and running ten 800s, each one in a slightly different dimension. Are we good?

HOW TO RUN IT

To run intervals in different dimensions, you need to adjust your pace based on the vibration frequency (VF). Obviously! For VF 1, run the 800 at your 10k pace. For VF 2, run half the 800 at 10k pace and half faster than 5k pace. For VF 3, divide the 800 into three parts: 10k pace, faster than 5k pace, 10k pace. Divide your VF 4 into four alternately paced parts, and your VF 5 into five parts. For the second set, run the VFs in reverse order, starting at 5. Also, reverse the way you alternate paces.

REST INTERVAL

30-second active rest between intervals; 2-minute active rest between sets

HERE'S WHERE IT HURTS

Intervals in a known dimension are hard. Switching dimensions while remembering frequencies and paces can tangle all thinking. During your second five dimensions, you'll either visualize a neat unified theory of everything or your dimensional insignificance will force you to seek shelter in the nearest porta potty.

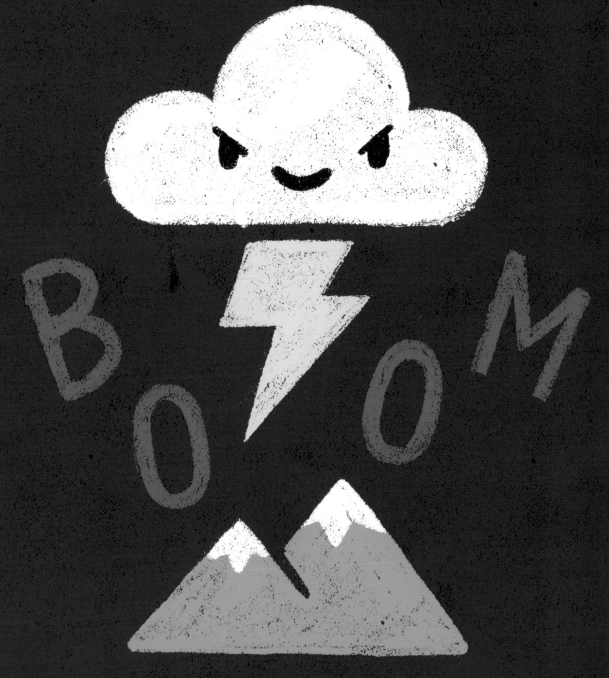

100% chance of PAIN

Mountaintop Lightning

DISTANCES: 2 x (200, 400, 800, 1200, 800, 400, 200)

- -

LUNG BURN:

Some of us love climbing mountains. Fresh air, beautiful views, communing with the natural world. Of course, upon setting out on a climb, you should always check the weather. It turns out getting struck by lightning isn't as unlucky as we've been led to believe. People get struck by lightning all the time, especially near high points like mountaintops.

We climb two mountains for this workout, and we've ignored the forecast. Running three shorter intervals gets you to the summit. Lightning strikes as you arrive at the viewpoint, so you sprint. As you circle the summit, the storm repeatedly zaps the ground around you, forcing a series of short sprints. The storm passes as soon as you descend into the trees. At the bottom, however, you decide to climb the mountain a second time without checking the weather. Runners never learn, do they?

HOW TO RUN IT

Run each of the shorter intervals at a steady 5k pace. During the 1200, lightning strikes every 100m forcing you to alternate between sprinting and running your 5k pace: Sprint the first 100m, run the 100m slower, sprint the third 100m, and so on.

REST INTERVAL

30-second active rest between intervals;
2-minute active rest between sets

HERE'S WHERE IT HURTS

To put a bright boltlike point on things, this workout includes a dozen 100m sprints intermingled with 5k running pace. Accelerating into your sprints during the second 1200 requires an Aconcagua fortitude you may not know you have.

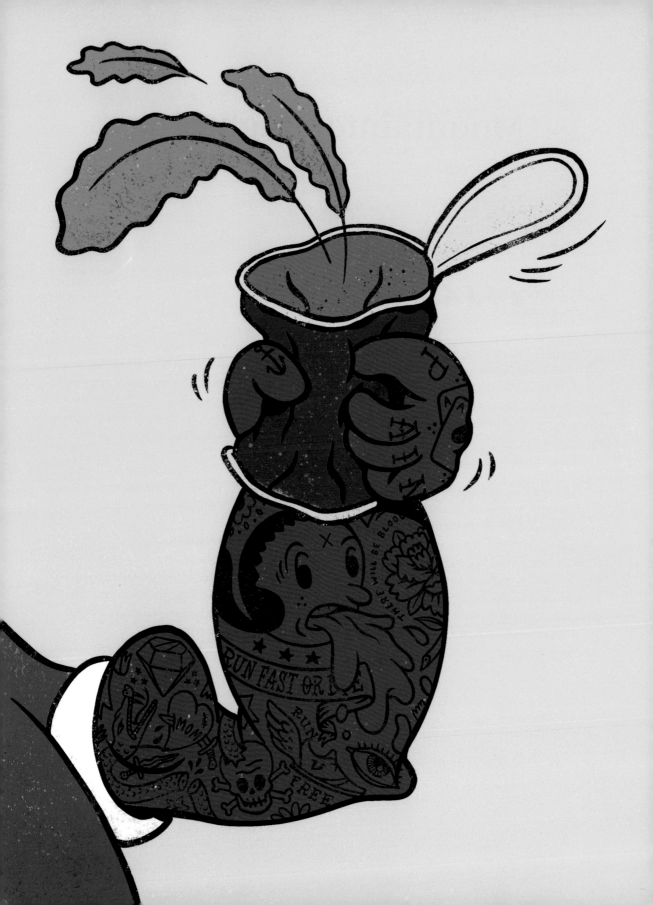

I Yam Popeye

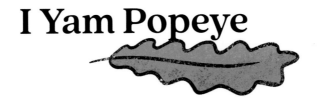

DISTANCES: 3 x 500, 3 x 800, 3 x 500, 3 x 300, 3 x 200, 3 x 300

- -

LUNG BURN: 🔥 🔥 🔥

Popeye, the sailor man who, by the way, didn't live in a garbage can but did come from modest beginnings, is famous for attaining superhuman strength immediately after chugging a can of spinach. Begin skinny and weak. Encounter bad guy. Shotgun canned spinach. Instantly sprout huge forearm muscles. Throttle bad guy. Pronounce "I'm strong to the finish 'cause I eats me spinach." That was his M.O., and it could be yours too. But let's just state for the record that canned spinach is disgusting, and anyone who's able to shoot it must be superhuman in some respect.

Turns out Popeye was indeed somewhat extra–human. The corncob pipe he smoked became a jet engine whenever he needed to augment his formidable forearms. So, like Popeye, this workout begins humbly and builds to an explosion of energy.

HOW TO RUN IT

We'll do a three-level progression within each interval set. Run the first interval at your 10k pace, the second somewhat faster, and the third at your 5k pace. Feel free to call out "I yam what I yam" after you finish the third interval in each set.

REST INTERVAL

10-second rest between intervals;
90-second active rest between sets

HERE'S WHERE IT HURTS

With only 10-second rests between the intervals within a set, the fast third 800 will push some pain buttons. The shorter intervals in the last three sets look doable until you factor in that short rest period. Bring the jet fuel in order to run strong to the finish.

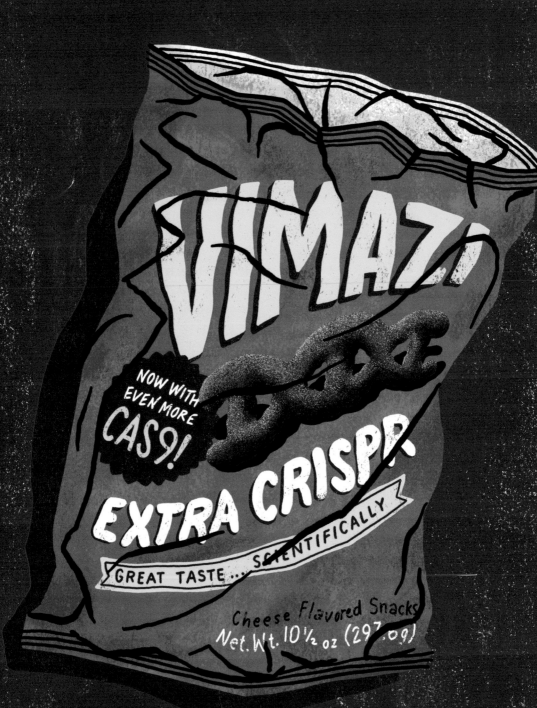

Prime Editing

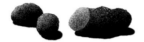

DISTANCES: 2 × (100-500-400-200, 1600, 200-400-500-100)

- -

LUNG BURN: 🔥🔥🔥🔥🔥

Prime editing, like CRISPR–Cas9 (page 78), is a gene editing technology that may be used by future molecular biologists. It's kind of like a biologist's search-and-replace feature. Exciting like the original CRISPR, only more so. Prime editing can locate DNA sequences and replace specific code. But rather than cutting the double helix, prime editing nicks the strand, allowing for code replacement in a more definitive way.

While CRISPR is used in a number of high-tech science labs for real-world applications, prime editing remains a proof of concept. Experimental? Unknown results? Possibility of spectacular failure? That's the sort of workout we like best.

HOW TO RUN IT

We'll run two prime editing sequences. Each sequence has a set of short search intervals, followed by a longer replace interval, then another set of short intervals. Run the short intervals fast and hard—faster than your 5k pace. Run the two 1600s steady at your 5k pace.

REST INTERVAL

10-second rest between the shorter intervals; 90-second active rest on either side of the 1600s; 2-minute active rest between sets

HERE'S WHERE IT HURTS

Okay, we're basically running 5 miles at or faster than your 3-mile race pace, with limited rest. If that sounds impossible to you, then you may want to skip to the next workout. But if you don't mind running into the unknown or puking up a couple lungs halfway through your second round of prime editing, then this might just be the workout for you.

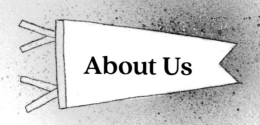

About Us

VIMAZI TRACK CLUB

We exist to champion the spirit of running. In addition to *Running in Circles*, we offer a free training app, *Vimazi RunCrush*, that creates a personalized daily mileage and pace plan focused on the goal you want to achieve. *Vimazi RunCrush* has a companion Apple Watch app as well. We also host an engaging series of virtual running events with themes based on illustrations from this book. Coming in 2021, look for Vimazi pace-tuned running shoes. You'll finally be able to run in a shoe that's built for your pace. Which makes sense in every dimension (p. 82). Get all the scoop at vimazi.com.

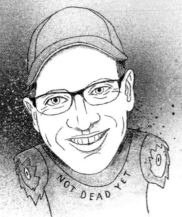

Scott Tucker, who became a serious runner during the 1970s streaking fad, spent his formative years at the altar of Douglas Adams and Monty Python. A physics degree led, naturally, to a career in running shoe design.

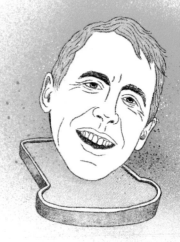

John Zilly parlayed a philosophy degree with a minor in collegiate cross-country into the writing of 10 mountain bike guidebooks and a deeply personal existential study of peanut butter and jelly sandwiches. Tucker and Zilly co-founded Vimazi.

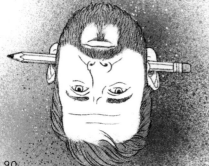

Jason Grube matriculated from running through the cow pie-filled pastures of central Wisconsin to, he much prefers, walking Pacific Northwest mountain trails and obsessively drawing pictures.